LIKE A NEEDLE IN A HAYSTACK

MY SURVIVAL FROM STAGE-4 PANCREATIC CANCER

By

Allison Kuban

with Sheldon Lippman

To my Uncle Sheldon who helped write this book
and bring this project to life.

To the nurses, doctors, hospital staff, and researchers
that took care of me and believed in me during my darkest days.

To the #RallyforAlli community and all my friends
who continue to lift my spirits.

To my parents and family who promised
I would never be alone and have always been by my side.

To my prince charming, Eric, for giving me purpose and life.

Thank You!

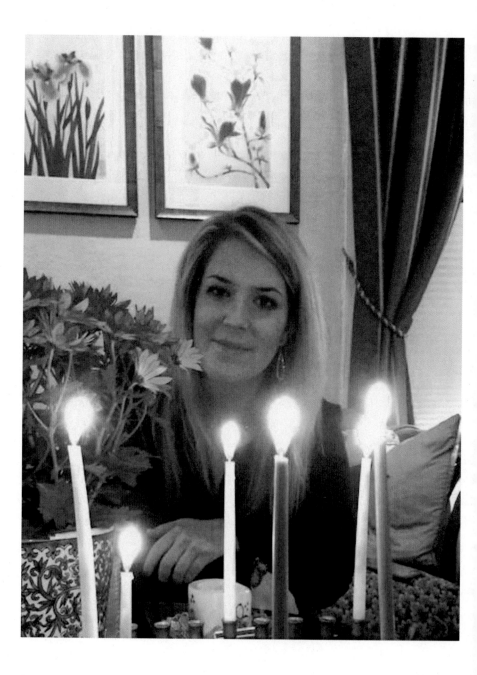

THIRTY AND FLIRTY

The pact that I declared for myself at 29½ years of age was simple...*no more dating until I turned 30 in June 2016.*

The birthday marking my third decade on Earth was quickly approaching, and I wanted to focus on me, myself, and I, with time for travel and other adventures; career and requisite job promotions; and maybe some new hobbies. Almost everything would be an option, except dating.

Admittedly, before the June 12 deadline approached and I would enforce my declaration, I had created an online dating profile and went on a few dates. One date was with a German guy who seemed really great until he told me he had a cat. Not just any cat, a hairless Sphynx cat. I hate to show my prejudices about pet cats, but basically this one looked like a raw chicken breast. My date just called it Kitty but I named it Tyson. We went on a second and third date. *Could I get past the fur-free feline?* As it turned out, after he kissed me on that third outing, I knew it was a bust. This was about the time that I thought long and hard about the dating scene and the approaching 3-0. I was not getting any pleasure from looking and trying. *Why the hell do I need a boyfriend?*

The life of a young professional is tough. We want to go out and have a social life but still need to work a 60-hour week to bust butt and establish a career. On top of that, add going to the gym, getting chores done, paying bills, engaging in community service (because that is what employers expect), getting the obligatory pedi-mani, having brunch with the girlfriends, weekend trips to see the family, and just keeping up one's appearance in general.

The hospitality industry caught my imagination as a teenager on a family vacation in Florida. I was in awe of the resort's general manager who walked around the pool area meeting with the guests. Being an impressionable teen, I could picture myself in a job walking around a luxurious pool talking to people from all over the world.

Carrying through with that career possibility, I enrolled in the hospitality program at Texas Tech University in Lubbock. I spent a semester at Apicius International School of Hospitality in Florence, Italy in their culinary and hospitality program. My first hotel job was in Park City, Utah. I returned to Texas for a short stint at a resort on Lake LBJ near Marble Falls and found more professional growth at a major hotel in College Station. By the time I was 26, I was climbing my way up the managerial ladder at a hotel in Dallas. My career path seemed well on its way; my dating life, no so much.

I admit to being part of the dating problem. My standards were too high. My sister-in-law Miranda told me I was too picky. Someone whom I dated once told me that I could never change a guy. *Was that a challenge?* I didn't think it was true, and I tried. It failed. I saw the light. You can't go on a first date thinking that you will be able to change this, that, or the other about someone. Some things may change with time; but you can't just ask a person to erase the sun tattoo around his nipple or ask a guy to adopt a furry kitten.

If I started to extrapolate a date into marriageable material, I had my dad as my exemplary benchmark. How could any man compare to my dad? My dad took me on dates when I was a little girl. We went to concerts, dinners and movies. He bought me flowers. Our first date was to Red Lobster and then a movie. On that first date, I had a Shirley Temple and got to take the glass home. That glass was the pen cup on my bedroom desk until I was 18 and went off to college. My dad was the gold standard by which I judged my dating prospects. *Sorry guys, big shoes to fill.*

As my 30ᵗʰ birthday approached, I made a decision in favor of personal growth and adventure. First big step, I would take myself on a trip to England to visit my cousins and several family friends. I bought the ticket, picked out my perfect outfits, and set myself up to take two weeks off from work. I had never taken two weeks off from any job since I started working after college. It was a big deal to ensure the hotel and my staff would be prepared for my extended absence. I would not be around for the midnight calls about unhappy guests or broken toilets. I was ready to embark on this life-changing trip that conjured up literary images of the book *Eat, Pray, Love* and I was the central character on an adventure.

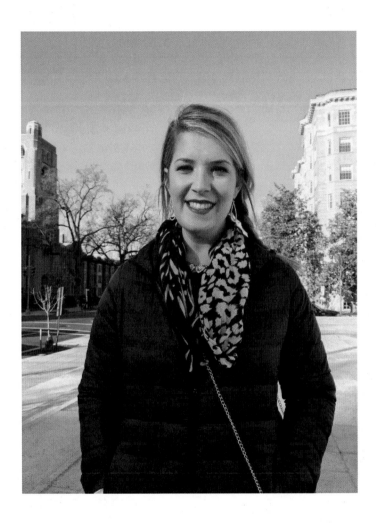

LONDON, HERE I COME

I was feeling liberated that April day in 2016 after the overnight flight to Heathrow Airport and looking smart in my new navy jumpsuit. Really, I felt pretty and confident in that jumpsuit except when I had to strip down in the lavatory every time I needed to pee. That was a small price to pay for looking and feeling great when I was greeted by my cousin Julia at the Hitchin bus station. It was not long after we arrived at Julia's flat in this quaint village that we sat down in her living room to begin chatting.

After more than an hour, we finally stood up for another activity. Much to

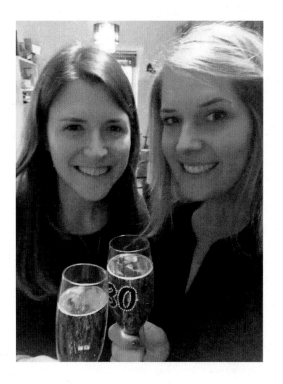

my horror, I had left a big blue mark the size of my bum on her lovely suede, beige couch. The blue of my new jumpsuit had rubbed off. When I went to shower and change clothes, I was shocked to see the bath towel was blue and my whole body had a tint of blue. I was turning into a blueberry-colored Oompa Loompa. Not quite the colorful impression I was hoping to make upon my arrival in England. Julia is a sweetheart. In spite of leaving my mark on her sofa and towels, she put me at ease and we had the best time chatting, cooking, and drinking bottomless bubbly. I saw other family and friends who entertained me all over London.

As a side trip from London, I flew to Spain with family friends and had the best week on the La Manga coast. I recall a moment of overlooking the cliffs and sea with the breeze in my hair and thinking *all was well in the world*. I had not yet turned 30, but if I could drink bottomless gin and tonics at a resort in Spain and feel this great, why would I need a man in my life. I was content. I was turning 30 and embarking on this new decade with my own goals and feeling g-o-o-d.

Traveling alone can be exhilarating. I was in touch with myself and felt my soul come to life. I hash-tagged everything with #eatpraylovetravel. It was the sum of everything I loved; I felt so proud, so confident, so ready to bring on 30.

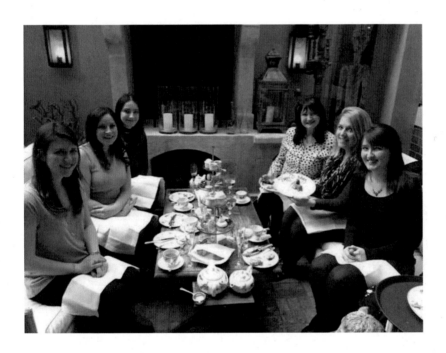

I HAD MY GOALS AND MY STANDARDS

When I returned to the States, I was scheduled to go to the corporate office of my hotel management company in Denver for an on-boarding meeting for new general managers. I had not officially been promoted, but they were grooming me for the next step. I was crossing things off my career bucket list and was happy and excited to embrace the potential promotion. I wasn't interested in baby steps. I wanted giant, bounding leaps forward.

Around this time, my mom called and said, "I gave your number to Betty for this guy to call you." Betty was a coworker of my mom and had a friend who wanted her son "to meet someone nice." Betty thought of me.

What?!? A guy calling me? This is so not in my plan. I had made it clear to myself that "this guy" cannot call until after June 12 when I turn 30. It was May so this guy is just going to have to hold off. Or maybe I'll ghost him and not answer if he calls. Information trickles in about this guy. He lives in the area. He is a pilot. He likes to travel.

Hold on, Allison, these are great qualities. Do you take the risk of going on a date? Or do you stick to the plan for self-loving contentment and remain on the self-driven path?

In the meantime, I was on the way back from the GM orientation when, low and behold, my phone rang. I knew this guy had my number from Betty. I answered the call. I didn't have time to really talk so I just politely explained I was returning from a work trip and would love to chat with him when I had more time. Besides, I was on a plane and my boss was sitting in front of me. Did I really need him ridiculing me for chatting with a guy as soon as we landed?

A few days passed when I realized I never called this guy back. I ghosted him, and I honestly didn't even mean to. However, an opportunity presented itself one weekend as I was driving between Houston and Dallas.

I decided I would give this guy a quick call in the car to kill time on the road. Maybe he wouldn't answer and I could just leave a voicemail.

He answered my call. I don't remember what we talked about. Somehow the Dallas skyline was quickly approaching as I realized we had been talking for over an hour. *What is happening?* I never have enough to say on phone calls, let alone for an hour, but we kept each other's attention. Time flew by quickly. This guy asked me out to dinner. I told him I could meet him on Monday evening.

IS THIS A DATE?

Monday, May 16, 2016, arrived. I could not think of any excuse to delay this date. *Date? Was this a date? Or was I just satisfying my mother's and Betty's urging?*

I left work early to go to the gym. I returned home to shower, change and meet this guy for the date. *Date? I am showered and dolled up. It's a date.* was about ten minutes from the restaurant, and he texted me, "I'm out front wearing a plaid shirt." I replied, "On the way. I'm wearing jeans, a black top, and have blonde hair."

This guy was waiting out front for me. We gave each other a cordial hug and walked into the restaurant. It was like I was meeting up with an old friend. I never had butterflies or felt nervous, just a calming sense of peacefulness. Everything felt just the way it should on a first date.

Wait! What is going on?

All that I remember is that I was enjoying myself and not over thinking or over analyzing this...date. A really nice date. Three hours went by with endless laughter and stories. When it was time to depart, we hugged and said "talk to you soon" and went our separate ways.

This guy is Eric. Eric Kuban. He is a pilot so his schedule is not the basic daily 9 to 5. He flies routes from New York to destinations along the East Coast. As days went by, we exchanged text messages to keep in touch. *Whoa!* I was feeling a rush in my heart every time I saw my phone light up with Eric's name, now plugged into my contact list. We arranged a second date that next weekend when he returned from his scheduled flights.

On Friday of the date-weekend, my parents came to visit me. We spent time exploring different neighborhoods, eating, drinking, and shopping. I nonchalantly told them I was supposed to go on a date that Sunday afternoon with the guy who Betty, my mom, and Eric's mom set me up with. My dad insisted that I had to go on the date and not to worry about being with them on Sunday. I really wasn't feeling any pressure from my parents, but when I tried on a dress that my dad ended up buying for me, he stipulated one rule...I had to wear it on my date.

TWO DOWN

Eric picked me up and we went to the Arboretum, a place I'd always thought would be perfect for a date. We walked around, talked, and had brunch. As we left the restaurant, his hand grazed mine and he held on to it. It felt comfortable. No sweaty palms. No awkwardness. When Eric dropped me off at my apartment, he got out of the car and came around to my side and hugged me. As I moved away, he leaned in and kissed me. Our first kiss, May 22, 2016. It was really romantic even though it took place next to the port-a-potty that was in a construction zone in front of my apartment.

Was this a sign? Eric and Allison make the most of any situation that life puts in front of them.

I can hardly believe what is happening. I am on cloud nine. When my parents grilled me about the date, I couldn't really put into words how I felt. My dad said, "I have a good feeling about this one." And, honestly, I did too.

Our budding relationship was easygoing and happening so naturally. The only odd thing was that Eric had to be away for long periods because of his job. We were putting to the test that adage, *distance makes the heart grow fonder*. It's so true. On the upside, I had so many plans for myself that our time apart allowed me to focus on work and achieve my personal goals. On the downside, I found myself missing him when he was away. I was eager to talk to him when he landed and called me. Never running out of things to talk about was nice. It was easy. Eric was becoming my new best friend.

IT ISN'T REAL UNTIL IT'S POSTED ONLINE

It was not very long after that first date, in early June 2016 that I was fantasizing about being Eric's girlfriend. He hadn't asked me to be his girlfriend. Eric wasn't on social media for me to make it FBO (Facebook Official), so I couldn't receive the friend request or any other virtual sign on social media that I was his girlfriend. But, dammit, I wanted it to be official.

I asked him if his parents knew about me. His reply was "baby steps." I was taking an opposite approach and telling the world about this new guy in my life. I couldn't wait to have my family meet him. They referred to him as "the pilot" and asked me on a daily basis: "When are we meeting the pilot? Is he your boyfriend? Where is the pilot now? When are you going out together again?" It was odd referring to Eric as my boyfriend since it was important to me that he should declare our relationship status. Someone had to get this fire started.

> Allison: "I won't be your girlfriend until you ask me."
>
> Eric: "Do people still do that?"
>
> Allison: "I don't care what people do. You need to ask me."
>
> Eric: "Will you be my girlfriend?"
>
> Allison: "I'll think about it. Just joking. Yes."

MEETING THE KUBANS

In early June, Eric made a weekend plan for me to meet his family. Eric's mother Cathy, father David, and brother Steven with his wife Kali greeted me with hugs and smiles like they knew me but hadn't seen me in a long time. We all went to lunch at a little café on a picturesque country road near his family's ranch outside of Glen Rose. Conversations flowed and stories were exchanged throughout the meal. Afterwards, we spent the afternoon at Leaning K, their ranch. The girls picked wildflowers while the guys tinkered in the barn.

The next weekend was my birthday, the big 3-0. My goal of not dating anyone had clearly failed. I couldn't imagine spending my birthday with anyone but Eric.

HAPPY BIRTHDAY TO ME

On the weekend of my birthday, June 12, Eric joined me on my planned weekend in Houston. We were staying at my brother Andrew's house while he and Miranda were at a wedding in San Diego. My parents were babysitting my two-year-old nephew, Jack. Eric and I had a day full of fun exploring antique shops and relaxing over afternoon drinks. The weekend was perfectly ordinary, a laid-back visit. Eric was fitting in perfectly with my parents and Jack.

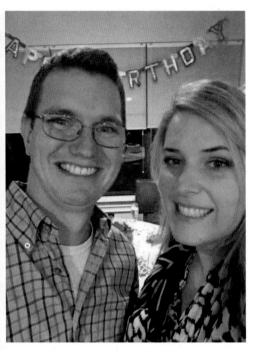

Eric and I stopped during our road trip to Houston to purchase sour candies to help Jack with his potty training. Much to my surprise, Jack quickly reached for "Uncle Eric's candy" instead of his typical two M&M's that he received when successfully using the potty. I couldn't wait to get Andrew and Miranda's approval of Eric, the next time we were together.

Eric had to leave on the morning of my birthday to do his piloting thing. I drove him to Bush Intercontinental early that day. As I was dropping him off, he gave me a homemade birthday card. The card was a huge pink foam flower with a selfie that we had snapped of the two of us on one of our first dates. It was so simple and childish and cutesy and silly, but the absolute sweetest, loveliest, most thoughtful thing I had ever received.

"Happy 30th Birthday, Babe"

My gosh. How disgustingly cute we were.

I think my heart skipped a few beats that weekend. As we said our goodbyes, I asked if I could make it FBO. *I mean, hello, it is 2016. If it's not on Facebook, it didn't happen.*

Presto Chango! Allison Lippman. In a relationship (with a picture). Happy effing 30th. Life doesn't go as planned. *Case. In. Point.* But, oh my gosh, I was happy!!!

Turning 30 wasn't so bad after all. I had Mr. Wonderful in my life. My career was still an important part of my identity. I had gone to school for hospitality management, moved across the country for jobs, met various goals on the career ladder, and basically lived and breathed my work. I was finally promoted to General Manager and who else would I want to celebrate with than my "official boyfriend?" For my promotion to GM, Eric made a handmade congratulatory card and bought flowers and a bottle of wine to celebrate. We were both career-driven and having someone who appreciated this meant so much to me. I was winning at life.

THOSE ALL-IMPORTANT THREE LITTLE WORDS

Our relationship continued to grow. Eric went with me on frequent visits to see my family during the summer. He still had his apartment in Fort Worth but was spending more and more time in Addison with me. Our evenings were full of conversation, drinks by the pool, dinners at home or new restaurants, and walks around the park. One particular clear summer evening, we went for a walk hand in hand in the park. Eventually we sat on a bench to enjoy the romantic sunset. We continued to talk, but I don't remember the gist of the conversation except the last three words from Eric, "I love you!"

Love. We had not mentioned the four-letter word up to this point. One month into the relationship and the feeling was mutual. I knew at that moment I could never love anyone the way I was falling for Eric. He made me want to live life to the fullest and made me want to seek every adventure that life had to offer. We quickly made the hashtag #adventuresofAandE for all our pictures. How perfect a beginning.

The lease at Eric's apartment was ending so we decided that he would move into my tiny apartment in Addison. This was a big step. I had never lived with a guy, so it was going to be quite an adventure.

My one-bedroom, 500-square foot apartment was adequate for me. I loved it dearly and had decorated it to my taste. But I had to accommodate. I moved a few things around in my closet so Eric was able to hang clothes, like two shirts. We went through his housewares to see what else we could cram into the kitchen cabinets. It was an exercise of shutting the doors and hoping nothing would fall out when opened. The A&E team made it work.

Eric brought a dresser from his apartment. I moved a few more things around. No problems were too big to solve. The cute shelf above the toilet that held my perfectly folded towels prevented the toilet seat from staying up while Eric went pee. The solution was that I allowed him to tie a bungee cord to the shelf so he didn't have to hold the seat up.

I was very particular about my space so allowing someone to make changes required a few extra glasses of wine and conversations that ended in our test-of-faith question we would always ask each other, "Do you love me more than an hour ago?" And of course, we did.

TRAVELING IS A TRUE TEST

Our adventures around Dallas continued from August to December 2016. I had booked a flight in December to visit my uncles, Sheldon and John, in Washington, DC. This was going to be their last Christmas in their DC home, Villa Veazey, before they moved to Austin. I was their first visitor when they purchased the house in 1999. I helped them to plan wall colors and visited their home many times over the years. I wanted to see their spectacular trademark Christmas decor one more time. I really wanted Eric to see it too. He was able to get a stand-by seat on the same flight. We spent a long weekend admiring the holiday spirit all over Washington and getting additional family approval of Eric.

As a pilot, Eric gets a Delta companion ticket for someone to share in his flight privileges. He still had his ex-girlfriend listed as his guest. Now he had someone new to add to this perk. Being the gentleman he was, Eric wanted

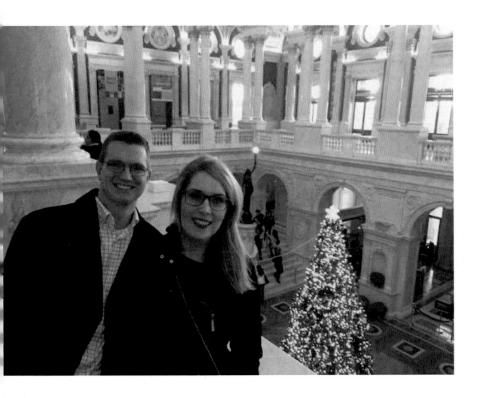

to give this ex advanced notice in case she wanted to use the pass one more time before he added "Allison Lippman" as his traveling companion.

There was still a mandatory waiting period before he could update the companion ticket with a new name. After about two months, Eric sent me an email with the documentation that I was now his traveling companion!!! We did not waste any time in planning our first international trip together.

IT IS ALL TOO ROMANTIC

April 2017, just one year since I had embarked on a solo trip to England and Spain, I was now with my boyfriend returning to Europe. I was with my boyfriend, the pilot. I was with my boyfriend, the pilot who got us upgraded to First Class. *Who am I? I can hardly recognize this girl.*

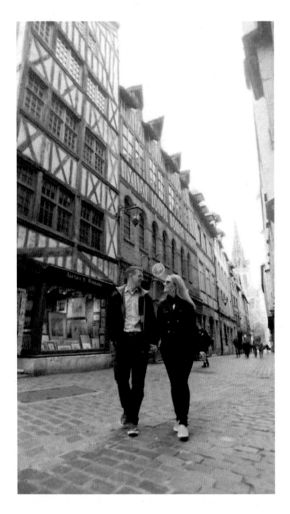

We had both been to France before. I went with my family when I was younger and had revisited in 2007 when I was studying abroad in Florence. It was different this time.

The trip was indescribable. France is absolutely beautiful and romantic and especially so with someone you love. Every little thing is more special. Every sip of wine explodes with flavor. Every macaron taste more desirable than your most favorite dessert. Every building or flower or park bench or

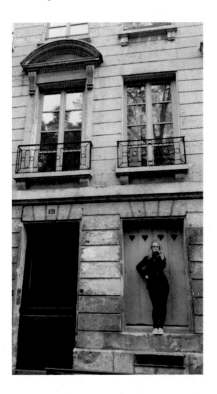 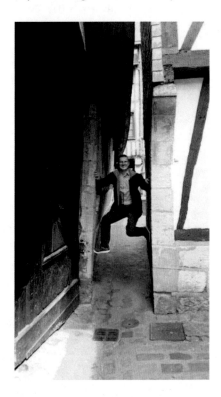

streetlamp is more spectacular than anything, anywhere. We spent the week driving through the French countryside, finding a charming hotel along the way, and exploring the nooks and crannies of the unfamiliar villages together. It was a different way to travel for me.

For my big 30th birthday trip to Europe, I had everything planned. Even that stupid blue jumpsuit. Usually, I travel with a big suitcase, a different outfit for every day, all my hotels planned out, and an itinerary to fill my time. In Eric's travel mode, I had one carry-on bag. I had fewer clothes but more freedom to live in the moment. We were spontaneous to explore each day as it comes and to revel in the unexpected. It was different from my travel experiences. Even if we did not know exactly where we were going, we were headed somewhere together.

Of course, my friends and family thought we were going to France to get engaged. This was not really on my agenda and I did not think it was on Eric's either. But he is good at surprises. I knew we would get engaged at

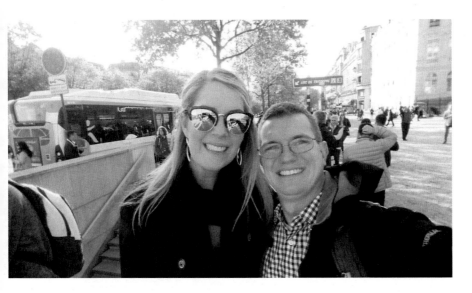

some point so I had given him five rules that he must follow before giving me an engagement ring:

1. Make sure my nails were done. (I did have them done for this trip. I mean, duh, who wouldn't?)

2. Make sure there is a photographer.

3. Use my full name when proposing.

4. Get on one knee.

5. Ask my dad. (Ok, this should be #1. I knew he had not met this yet.)

Honestly, there was part of me that was still hopeful. We had the perfect setting. We had been together for almost a year. Oh well, it didn't happen in Paris, France. I wasn't disappointed but was excited. Where would he pop the question if not in the most romantic city in the world?

TOO MUCH OF A GOOD THING, OR NOT SO GOOD

Eric and I were back to reality in Dallas with busy schedules. We returned home on a Thursday and headed to see Eric's family for the annual Granbury Wine Walk. It wasn't exactly what I had in mind considering I was jet lagged and had just drank a fair share of spectacular wine in France.

We walked from booth to booth and I was incredibly hot and tired, unable to drink the wine, and feeling border-line sick. I had a pain in my left side and was uncomfortable. I figured I was just beyond tired and couldn't wait to get into air conditioning, lay in bed, and sleep.

I went back to work on Monday and dove immediately into writing the mid-year sales review. I was stressed, tired, and just wanted to go back to France. I would look through the pictures on my phone to reminisce of the many special moments of the most amazing trip; then refocus and quickly get back to work. But, like a bombshell, my left side hurt worse than ever. I breathed through the pain, which would subdue to a point that I could return to work on the sales review.

For most of the following month I figured my body was going through withdrawal or detoxing after drinking and eating such rich and gorgeous food and wine throughout the trip. The pain would come and go. I convinced myself that it was a good thing that my body was undergoing a spontaneous cleansing and trying to normalize itself. I was starting to see my weight drop and my appetite dwindle. I thought maybe I had a gluten intolerance. Dairy intolerance? Meat? Alcohol?

I wanted some explanation for every sharp pain I felt in my side. I spoke with Eric's dad, who is an internal medicine physician, hopefully to shed some light on the issue that was consuming not just my body but my life. David recommended various medicines to treat whatever gastrointestinal symptoms I was enduring. These recommended medicines changed frequently as my symptoms kept multiplying. The colon spasm pills in particular became my talisman. Like a lucky charm, I did not leave home without them. I took them before, after, and during my meals. However, it wasn't working. The pain continued to hit me like a ton of bricks.

Since the pain was not on my right side, I could eliminate the appendix or gallbladder. But then I would think that maybe the pain was so severe that it was being directed to other places in my body, like my left side. This is where my head was at; diagnosing myself, explaining and rationalizing the pain. I concentrated on my diet in case it was food related. I eliminated bread. Eric kept me accountable and would take away any starch from me as a precaution.

With both of my parents in the medical field, I would text my mom and dad with every new and recurring symptom to see what they thought. Their educated guesses were becoming exhausted. They suggested I meet a doctor for further investigation. Enough was enough. I booked an appointment with an internal medicine doctor whom my aunts in Dallas referred me to. Of course, the pain had subdued the day I visited this doctor. Still, she booked a CT scan for that afternoon to take a closer look at what was going on.

I continued staying busy at work and was stressed. I was stressed from work, stressed from my body attacking me, stressed that I couldn't exercise, stressed that I couldn't stand up to cook dinner, and especially stressed that I couldn't enjoy my time with Eric.

A few days later, I went in for my follow-up appointment. The responses from this appointment were bewildering. "We couldn't see anything, so I think it is stress or anxiety with everything you are facing at work. Maybe you should take Prozac to help control these symptoms." There was more. "There are a few spots on your liver, but again, it's nothing to worry about." I walked out with my report. *What the hell? Am I crazy? Prozac?* I told my dad and he said, "No! There are too many side effects with Prozac and you don't need to compound the problem." I looked over my report and saw the word "mass" and figured the doctor would have told me if it was something significant. She referred me to a GI specialist. I had an appointment for the following week. *Great, another week of hell.*

I carried on until my next appointment while Eric was away flying. I went back to the hotel and worked on my report and filled in on shifts, all the while fighting through the pain. At the breakfast shift one morning, I literally doubled over in pain at the cash register with every stab in my stomach that went through my back, up my spine, and pounded through my head.

The day of my appointment with the GI doctor finally came and Eric was with me. After waiting in the screening room, "Dr. Mark Ruffalo" entered. That is not really his name, but he reminded me of the actor. He was so cute! *Damn, and this man wants to talk about my bowel movements.* Of course, the pain had gone away that day as well, but I explained my symptoms.

Then *POW!* In a flash, a stabbing pain hit in front of cute "Dr. Ruffalo." I was sweating. He saw that there was something wrong and recommended that I book a colonoscopy as soon as possible. The appointment was made for the next week. I came out to the reception area where Eric was waiting for me. I told him that the doctor was wonderful and my colonoscopy appointment was next Thursday. "What? Next week?" fumed Eric, uncharacteristically frustrated. "Another week. That's bullshit. You can't wait another week!" What could I say except that we would have to wait another week.

As the next few days passed, the pain came and went but soon became more constant and lasted longer. I would sleep 12 to 14 hours as my body battled each stab. I called the doctor and asked that if any time becomes available before next Thursday, to please let me know, "I'm desperate."

Desperation puts it mildly. I was literally crippled over in pain trying to get through a workday. I was preparing for a big presentation at work. Who joyfully counts down the days until having a colonoscopy? That was me.

GOING OUT OF MY MIND AND OUT OF MY BODY

On June 5, the morning of the presentation at work, despite a rough weekend of enduring pain, I was so ready to have this performance over with, get the colonoscopy, and finally know what was going on inside my body. Mike, my hotel's regional vice president, knew of my medical situation since I had explained to him why I had to leave early for doctor's appointments or go home and sleep the pain off. I went to the office early that Monday morning to prepare the meeting room and get things ready for the presentation.

Erin, the regional sales vice-president, was sitting in a café booth eating her breakfast. I walked up to say good morning, dripping in sweat, light headed from the pain, and just hoping and praying for all this to pass so I could get through the day. On top of all else planned that day, Erin and I had scheduled an interview that morning for a new Director of Sales, a position that I desperately needed to fill.

Erin briefed me on the candidate, a well-dressed, older man, with an impressive resume. I glazed over the words on the piece of paper in front of me. I listened to Erin ask a question, then I looked at him for his answer. He spoke, but I heard nothing. All I could hear in that moment was me telling myself not to pass out. His answers were long. I just prayed for his mouth to stop moving, but he seemed to go on and on. I closed my eyes with each stab and just thought *mind over matter, mind over matter*. I'm sure if Erin had looked at my face, she would have known that I wasn't mentally in that room. The man, who no doubt wanted to make a good impression on the woman who could not look him in the eyes, wanted the job so bad.

When it was my turn to ask him a question, I couldn't form a coherent thought. I was out of my mind with pain. I just wanted to make it to the "thank you, we'll be in touch" so I could go home, lay down in the air conditioning, and breathe through it.

The interview ended. I shook his hand and he left. "I honestly was so absent from this interview," I said to Erin. "My mind was elsewhere." She understood and saw how much I was struggling. She sent me home and advised me to go to the ER if it got worse. "But what about my presentation?" She said it didn't matter and she would conduct training with the team since everyone was new to their position and desperately needed some guidance. I was never more thankful to leave the office.

I didn't think I could drive home in this much pain, but I managed to drive the five minutes to my apartment. I barely crawled up the stairs, got in bed, and prayed. I prayed that the pain would give me a break for an hour so I could sleep. I prayed for Eric to come home and take care of me. I prayed I could make it to Thursday for my colonoscopy. And I prayed I would not have to go the ER.

I always thought going to the ER was so over-dramatic, a last resort that meant you really are so sick that you need immediate life-saving attention. I laid in bed, feeling like I was sinking. Drowning in sweat, I was so light-headed on the verge of passing out. I probably did pass out because I woke up to my phone ringing. My dad called to ask me how the presentation went. When I told him that I didn't do it because I was in too much pain and was sent home, he went into dad mode and asked for the doctor's name and phone number. He said that I needed the colonoscopy now. I was so embarrassed and didn't want him calling and bothering the doctor when I had already asked to be moved up on the schedule. But he did call and left a message. He also called Eric to come home as soon as he landed at DFW and take me to the ER. My mom was in Houston where she was visiting Andrew, Miranda, and their month-old baby, my new nephew Ben. However, she left for Dallas later that evening.

Eric called when he landed and was on his way to pick me up to go to the ER. Of course, at that point, the pain was passing. I hopped in the shower to rinse off the sweat and then crawled back into bed. I kept telling myself that I was strong and could get through this.

My pilot, my hero, came to my rescue. Without a minute to catch his breath, Eric grabbed my pillow and helped me to the car for the drive to the hospital. I walked in on my own. The pain had subdued as I checked myself in feeling completely ridiculous that I should be considered an emergency case. It was only a matter of time when I was happy to be in a place that could identify the source of my misery.

An hour or more went by before I met with a nurse in the ER. They wrote down my symptoms and took my vitals. The hospital collected my insurance co-pay before I was led to a room. They hooked me up to an IV and gave me pain medicine to keep me comfortable. Eric was in the room with me. They told me they wanted to run some tests. I explained that I had a CT scan a few weeks ago and was told nothing was found; and a colonoscopy was scheduled for later that week. A nurse came in to take me to get an ultrasound while Eric stayed in the room.

I could tell he was nervous as he pulled out his phone every few minutes to text, play his numbers game, or look at me any time I flinched. *Was it only one month ago that Eric and I were in France?* We had celebrated our one-year dating anniversary just a few weeks earlier. Little did we know that we were about to embark on our next adventure.

When I returned from the ultrasound, my mom, who had just arrived from Houston, was in the room with Eric. The doctor came in and asked about my CT scan results from the weeks prior. I explained that I had the scan in the hospital, that the results didn't show anything, and I was told to take Prozac. He looked perplexed. He wanted to find the images and notes from the doctors who performed the CT scan. My ultrasound, he said, showed lesions in my liver. He wanted to keep me overnight for more testing the next day. *Lesions?* I looked to my mom who said, "Let's do the tests tomorrow and see what they say."

It was quite late in the evening at that point. We were all tired and ready to get settled. I was wheeled upstairs to a new room, where I crawled into the bed and laid down thinking about lesions. *What are lesions? Small cuts? Maybe I drank too much wine in France?* My mom called my dad from the

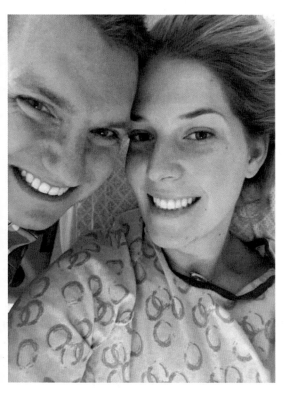

hallway. Eric held my hand with tears in his eyes. I was ready to sleep. In my half-dozing state, I thought I had to be strong for them, that it's okay. We will do the tests in the morning and go from there. *Why was Eric crying? I've never seen him cry or show any fear.* My mom stayed with me overnight so Eric could go home to get some rest. I must have fallen asleep with questions playing in my mind like a lullaby. *Lesions? Why was my boyfriend crying? Why did my mom call my dad to come to Dallas to be with us?*

The next morning, I was taken to radiology for a biopsy. My mom works in radiology from time to time at the hospital in Bryan, so I know it was surreal for her that I was the patient getting the biopsy. If she had any fear, it is beyond me how she hid it. She was so strong and at ease as I was drugged and wheeled out of the room. I had been told that they were taking a biopsy of my liver because it was easier to reach. I don't remember much from the procedure except feeling very light-headed as I was being wheeled back to my room and trying to get back into my bed. Time during that episode remains a blur.

Later that day, my dad was with me. It was unbearable seeing his tears and despairing for him to not have any answers for me at that moment. The pain in my heart hurt worse than the pain in my side. I thought the lump in my throat was going to kill me. In the midst of feeling so weak and desperate, I was so comforted to know my rock and #1 fan was there.

My dad messaged me:

> *I can't stop crying. I thought the tears would end, but they keep coming. I told Andrew to come to Dallas but couldn't say much more before I started crying. He is very upset and wants to see you.*

Andrew, Miranda, and Ben were on their way from Tomball to Dallas. Ben wasn't even a month old. When Ben was born, I didn't think I could love another nephew like I loved Jack. Jack was 3 years old at the time and was the absolute light of my life. I love being his Auntie Alli. I love every move, every look, every kiss, every word that Jack spoke. My heart was so full when I first saw Jack. But as soon as I met Ben, I adored him. I was so excited to see him, even in the hospital while hooked up to dripping and beeping machines, with no strength to walk more than five feet.

I was drowsy after the biopsy and with the various pain medicines. Having not left my bedside, Eric constantly reminded me that he was always going to be there for me. Cathy and David came from Granbury to see me. In fact, my hospital room was like Grand Central Station with visits from Eric's cousin, some of my friends and hotel staff, my aunts, and my GI doctor, the one who looked like Mark Ruffalo.

Although most of those visits remain a blur, I remember Andrew walking into the room and collapsing on my chest. I could feel his tears rolling onto my shoulder and him trying to catch his breath in between crying and trying to say, "I love you" and "You're going to be OK."

Next at my bedside was Miranda, who was still healing from having a baby just a month earlier and in the midst of getting a newborn's feeding schedule down, nurturing a three-year old, and being a loving wife to my brother. She hugged me with repeated assurances of "I love you." Miranda has an incredible way of making a person feel genuinely loved. I felt so lucky at that time to have such a strong person by my side.

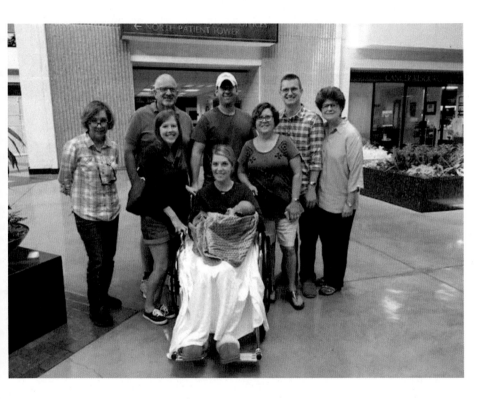

Ben stayed downstairs with my Aunt Marilyn since he could not be brought onto the oncology floor. *Oncology floor?* I had not heard that I was on the oncology floor until my mom left her phone on my bedside table when she went to the bathroom. I snooped and saw that she had texted a friend "Alli is on the oncology floor, but they haven't told her."

I wanted to see Ben. If he couldn't come to me, I would go to him. Eric and my mom helped me into the wheelchair and took me downstairs. I was incredibly weak but loved looking into Ben's eyes, and knowing I had to find the strength somewhere to cradle him and to get the hell out of this hospital to be Auntie Alli. To be Eric's girlfriend. To be a sister. To be a daughter. To get back to work. I was quickly feeling lost in an unfamiliar world.

WHAT IF THIS PAIN IS JUST CANCER

Without any real answers, I vaguely remember joking with Eric, "Oh my gosh, what if all this pain is just cancer?" We laughed at the absurdity, "I probably have IBS or something with my GI." I would just pop another one of those spasm pills.

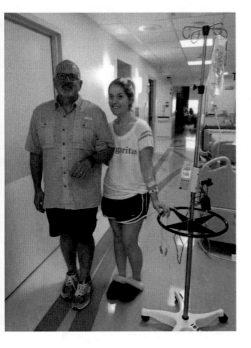

After three days in the hospital bed, I had reached my limit and was able to get up and hold onto my dad and walk up and down the hallways. My dad, who taught me to walk, to skip, to ride a bike, was holding up my weak body. I also walked with Eric to relieve the air in my belly from the biopsy that was causing horrendous hiccups. Eric had my hand just as he had when we walked the streets of charming French villages just a few weeks earlier. We never imagined this adventure down a hospital corridor.

During my naps, Eric went back to our apartment to shower and gather a few necessities for me, like a change of clothes and a toothbrush. He would grab a nap as he was completely exhausted, both physically and emotionally. One time when he wasn't by my bed when I woke up, I got upset. A few minutes later, he walked in the room with a huge green vase full of flowers. He apologized for being late but needed to get flowers for the vase. White lilies.

He was so sweet and I was so mad at myself for being impatient. My frustration level was reaching its peak. I was ready to leave the hospital, go back to work, live a normal life, and put my new green vase in the perfect spot in our apartment.

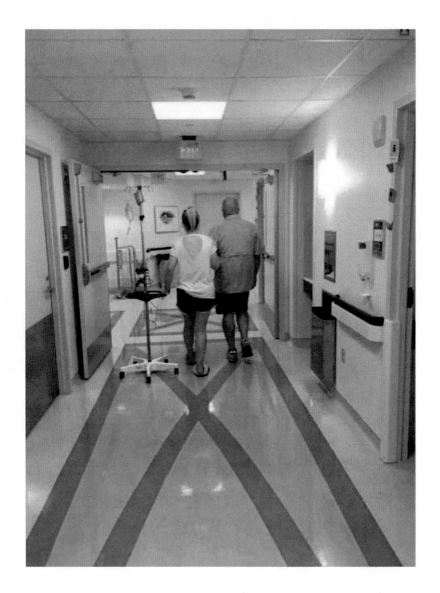

I asked Eric if he had gone to Pier One to get the vase. "No," he said, "I found it in the trash room of our apartment building." No joke, he was telling the truth. Eric will turn trash into treasure. If only he could turn me back into my old self. I felt helpless. Eric was measuring my urine after I used the bathroom each time to give to the nurse. He was helping feed me. He was sleeping in a recliner as I laid in my hospital bed. He constantly reminded me that he loved me and we would get through this together. I was his treasure.

"Take everything one exit at a time." That was the phrase Dr. Suresh, the floor doctor, would say when he gave us a piece of new information. On this particular morning, Dr. Suresh came in my room with the oncologist and said he was 90% sure of the diagnosis and was waiting on the final scans. That's all we could do.

Dr. Suresh asked my parents and Eric to talk with him in the hallway. That made me angry. *Just tell me what the hell is going on.* When they were still in the hallway, "Dr. Anonymous," the oncologist, had come in to discuss my diagnosis. He was impatient when I asked for him to wait until my family was in the room. He explained that I had neuro-endocrine cancer. I would need to take a hormone shot once a month. He recited this diagnosis and prescription with no emotion, which seemed cold to me. I guess he has to be more stoic when he gives patients a diagnosis such as this. *One exit at a time!*

Dr. Suresh and "Dr. Anonymous" left the room and I was alone with my parents and Eric. We were relieved that I would only require a monthly shot. I asked what their conversation was about in the hallway and was told that it was regarding all the medicines I needed to take and insurance. Things that I shouldn't be worrying about. Thank God I had my family with me. I had Eric. I had so much to be thankful for.

NOT THE WISH I WOULD BLOW OUT CANDLES FOR

It was Friday morning, June 9. I had been in the hospital for five days and was finally strong enough to be released. The nurse allowed me to pull out my own IV and get into the wheelchair. As I was being wheeled to

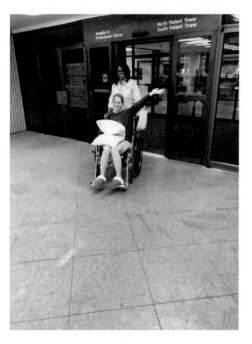

freedom, my dad was recording the hallelujah moment when I put my hands in the air and cried.

Since it was my 31st birthday weekend, my parents had already planned to come to Dallas. Instead of going on my planned itinerary around Dallas for cocktails, shopping, brunch, and fun, we hung out in our shoebox of an apartment. It's funny how life has so many plot twists when you try to plan it all out.

On Monday, June 12, my birthday, we sat around the apartment. Everyone sang happy birthday to me and I wore a birthday headband that my mom bought me. It wasn't the most ideal birthday, but I was happy to be home and out of the hospital. I was still weak and groggy, so naps were my jam.

The phone rang as I was preparing to take one of my birthday naps. I answered. It was "Dr. Anonymous." "Hi Allison, the remainder of your tests came in and the diagnosis has changed. Is there any way you and your family could come in this afternoon?" My heart sank. "Of course, they are still here because it is my birthday today." He said, "Oh, we can wait until tomorrow then." I responded, "No, I won't be able to enjoy the rest of my day with the anxiety of not knowing what is going on. We will come in."

I went into the living room and told my parents and Eric what the doctor said. Eric immediately called his mom and asked her to come to Dallas as he did not have a good feeling. That afternoon, we piled into the car and headed back to the hospital. We found our way to the office and checked in. All the while, I was answering texts, Facebook messages, and phone calls from my friends who were making me feel loved on my birthday.

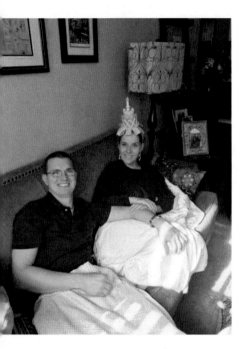

"Dr. Anonymous" came into the room and told us that the remainder of the scans came back and while they were about 90% sure, the scans showed a different result. "Allison has acinar cell carcinoma. It shows up in about 1% of pancreatic cancers. The pain is coming from the tumor wrapped around the splenic artery."

I was speechless. I was absolutely dumbfounded looking around the room at everyone. "A rigorous chemotherapy treatment needs to be started." *Chemo?* I asked the doctor if I would lose my hair. "Yes, after the second treatment it will start to fall out." *What is going on?* Life just made a drastic wrong turn on that so-called "one exit at a time." My bald head flashed in my mind. My dreams of marrying Eric were now at stake. *What about having kids after chemotherapy? How would this effect my body for years to come? Is there even a future to worry about?*

As a treat to myself during my birthday week, I had made a hair appointment. When I got home from that doctor's visit, I called the salon to cancel my appointment. "I was just diagnosed with cancer and I'm going to lose my hair so I need to cancel my appointment." I'm sure they didn't need any excuse or want to hear it. But I was angry and I had to say it. I had to say it out loud for the first time, "I have cancer!"

I began to let my friends know what was going on. It was hard to explain, but I had to remain positive. I had to remain strong. I had to remain thankful. I was happy it was me getting a diagnosis of this nature instead of Eric or my family. But, at that time, I had not fully appreciated that they were the ones who would suffer over the months ahead as I endured chemotherapy and a daily pill-popping regimen.

My friend Malori posted on Facebook and shared with many friends:

> As I'm writing this post, I feel like I need to have all of the perfectly right and eloquent things to say to express this, but sometimes the things that happen in life are not so right and eloquent, so I will just write...Our sweet Alli Lippman has had quite a difficult week this past week. She was put in the hospital for some terrible stomach pains and symptoms that have worn her body out. The most recent diagnosis came to her yesterday (on her birthday of all days!!!) which is that she has a rare form of pancreatic cancer. As with everything, she has taken this with such strength and positive optimism, and she hopes everyone will keep these positive thoughts with her as well! I am in shock and angry and find this just so unfair for something like this to happen to someone like this. However, unsurprisingly, during my conversation with her this evening, she just repeatedly kept saying how thankful she was for the prayers and love she had been getting already and said she already feels it. I also found out that she was checking up on others who have been going through some rough things right now...WHILE SHE WAS IN THE HOSPITAL! If all of that isn't a true sign of how much of a selfless and beautiful human being she is, I don't know what is. GOD AND HER BEAUTIFUL SPIRIT WILL BEAT THIS...SHE WILL BEAT THIS!!! As she begins chemo next week, anytime that you can think to take a minute, please pray for our amazing friend Alli! We believe in the power of prayers...as does she 100%!!!

Miranda asked if they could post something on social media. Of course, I said it was okay. Before long, she and Andrew created a Facebook group and shared:

As some of you may know, Alli has been sick for the past few weeks. On Monday, her 31st birthday, she was diagnosed with a rare cancerous tumor on her pancreas and liver. This news was obviously very devastating to her and the family, and we have struggled to make sense of it all. The encouraging news is that a treatment plan has been set and should begin in the near future. Unfortunately, the plan will involve a chemotherapy regime which will occur every other week for the next few months. At that point, the doctors will perform another scan and hopefully be cancer free! Alli is a very strong person and we know that she will come out of this even stronger. She has already received a tremendous amount of love and support, and we hope to keep that going throughout her treatment. Please keep Alli, her boyfriend Eric, and the rest of the family in your thoughts and prayers during this difficult time. I look forward to sharing some encouraging and positive news in the months to come! #RallyforAlli

My phone blew up. I received the most thoughtful and touching messages, notes, flowers, cards, letters, and calls from family, friends, people I didn't

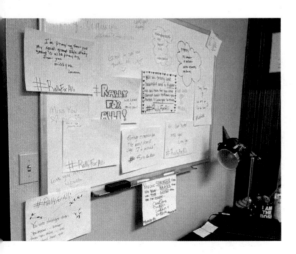

know very well and others who I thought had forgotten me over time.

Andrew and Miranda asked on Facebook for friends and family to send a picture with them holding a sign that said "Rally for Alli" to put on my wall in the living room. Miranda made a banner and my wall quickly filled up.

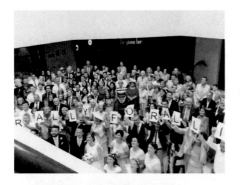
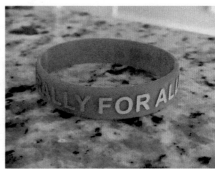
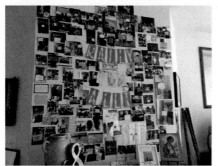
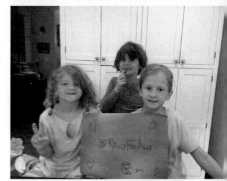
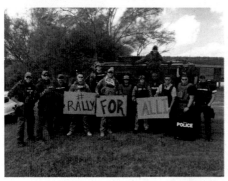
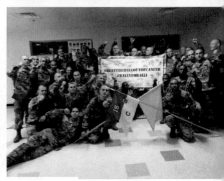
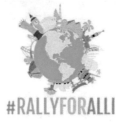

#RALLYFORALLI

WHEN YOU THINK YOU ARE DYING, GET A SECOND OPINION

On June 20, I was scheduled to get a port placed in my chest. My mom took me to the hospital that morning. Eric was in training but constantly called to check on me. My dad called to check on me and said that he would drive to Dallas when he was off work to be with me. The sweet nurse who started the IV said, "You are too young to be in here for this, but you're going to beat it. I just know it." I was quickly drugged up again and wheeled back for the procedure. *Procedure?* A procedure is a root canal or a colonoscopy, a quick and simple little thing that gets you in and out within the hour.

I was being set up for a procedure that would be a recurring bump on this crazy, winding highway of life. It was that "one exit at a time" on this journey ahead. My port was placed in my chest and secured with surgical tape. The port would leave a scar on my tan and freckled from the sun chest. Now I wanted to hide my scarred chest. However, my blouse or shirt would reveal the bump above my right breast. *I had a port. I was sick. I was dying.* For the first time since the diagnosis, I was feeling sorry for myself.

Days turned into weeks. I had the diagnosis. I had the port. The word was out. I was ready to start chemo. I had a social media presence. Facebook readers relayed their family cancer stories: someone's mom's aunt's friend's sister had pancreatic cancer. And I got advice. One of the best pieces of advice was from my friend who lost his wife to colon cancer. He said, "Get a second opinion."

As we all left "Dr. Anonymous's" office with a sour view of his bedside manner, we agreed that a second opinion was needed. Eric's dad mentioned my diagnosis to a fellow physician acquaintance who directed me to an oncologist at UT Southwestern in Dallas.

Eric was in training, so I went to that appointment with my parents and David. My friend, Jaime, who was a physician's assistant at UT Southwestern, had seen my story on Facebook and reached out to me. He had also encouraged me to come there and was excited to join me at my upcoming appointment. Jaime has the most amazing faith; so inspiring, so

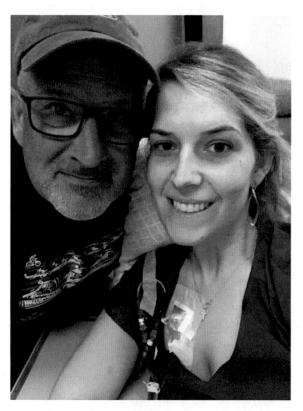

motivating, so hopeful. However, I could see the fear in his eyes when he came to say a prayer with us before the doctor came into the room.

My stars were aligned as I went to this first appointment with the new team. Enter Dr. Beg. He shook everyone's hand, sat down with his back to my family, and talked to ME. Talking eye-to-eye with Dr. Beg was a striking contrast from the previous oncologist who stood over me, barking out my diagnosis and my treatment plan; he showed no tact when he mentioned that my hair was going to fall out. His entire interaction with me did not show a lick of empathy. This lack of bedside manner did not go unnoticed. Now, with his focus on me, Dr. Beg explained that he had seen my scans and agreed with the diagnosis and explained the different stages of cancer. That's when I heard the stage-4 rating because the cancer had metastasized.

In a flash, I was no longer worried about when my hair was going to fall out. Now, my question was, "How long do I have to live?"

Dr. Beg did not know the answer. No one could answer that question. A question that was certainly not easy for parents to hear a child ask. Dr. Beg left our meeting, and his nurse, Viviana, came in to explain the next steps. I loved her name. She was tall, tan, calm and had long hair. Each word from her mouth was spoken softly as she explained the patient portal, support groups, and where to go for treatments. Her spirit, her aura, her nature were beautiful to my eyes despite the nature of the information. She had a calming effect. I may have been in a trance. She encouraged us to go to the support group meeting that was taking place that afternoon. As we started to walk down the hall to the meeting, the trance state disappeared. I broke down and collapsed crying. I told my dad that I couldn't talk to complete strangers when I just received this news ten minutes ago. We snuck into an unoccupied room and all cried. I sat between my mom and dad, "You are never alone. You will never do this alone. I want to take this from you. You can't go before me. One exit at a time." My hero was telling me, "You can't die before me."

We left the hospital and I called Eric to tell him what my diagnosis was. I told him how much I loved the nurse and doctor and wanted to proceed with them. My dad compared UT Southwestern to MD Anderson and knew I was supposed to be there. At that point, those "exits" were flying by. I was driving 100 MPH with a blindfold down the highway of life, ready to crash. I wanted to crash and wake up from this nightmare. But it was my new reality. My life was forever changed.

THE JOURNEY OF A LIFETIME

It was the next day when I started chemo. My parents drove me to a clinic in Richardson, which was closer to my apartment. It was also smaller and less overwhelming for my first treatment. That morning, I brought my pillow, a blanket from my beloved boss, my bag full of medicine, my binder where I tracked my doses, my phone, my charger, and my slippers. I was like an infant who needed a diaper bag of stuff to go anywhere. It was nearly three weeks since my stay in the hospital. I was embarking on a new journey...the next exit.

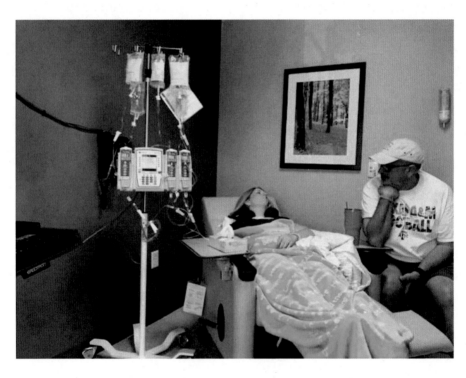

As I walked toward the clinic, I broke down. Crying, I looked at my parents, "This is my life now. This is your life now. Your daughter has cancer." I was mad. Not for myself, but for them. They were supposed to go to Spain that summer. The friends who I had visited in Spain for my 30th birthday were getting married. Instead, my parents were canceling their trip, trying to get a refund, trying to get a leave from work, and spending their time with me in Dallas. They should have been in Houston with my nephews, their grandsons. I was supposed to be working as a general manager at my hotel with a handsome boyfriend who had just gotten his dream job with Delta Air Lines.

Eric could not be with me on this day. He was training in Atlanta for his new job that he had worked hard for long before he met me. He could never have imagined this nightmarish scenario that faced him at home as he was learning to fly a new jet. In between his training sessions and on his breaks, he would call and check on me and say, "I love you." I was speechless. I was scared.

At the clinic, the port was accessed through the fresh, unhealed incision on my chest. I held my dad's hand as the nurse told me to take a deep breath as she pinned me. A few meds were administered, including a few drugs to help me relax before the chemo started. I slept through most of the treatment and chatted with Eric whenever he called or texted me. I looked at the flood of messages of encouragement on Facebook. The Rally for Alli page was filled with motivational quotes, messages, and pictures that I looked at over and over again.

Danielle, one of my friends that I met when I worked in Orlando during a college internship, shared several messages with me. She had been battling breast cancer for the last year and was a great resource for me during the initial days of my diagnosis. I could ask her questions like does your hair just fall out in one day or is it a process? I could tell her I was scared and she could confide in me what her trials and triumphs were. I was happy to have a message from her on the first day of my treatment.

Danielle: Hey Alli, just checking in on you and see how you are doing?

Alli: Hey girl! I start chemo today. It wasn't as good of an outlook as I hoped for but I'm still determined to fight and get it managed. It won't be cured forever but managing it is my goal. I can deal and live with that. Of course, hearing I'll be on chemo forever sucks, but I just have to take it one day at a time. If I start to think about my hair, or the future that I thought I was going to have (marriage, children, traveling), I get overwhelmed. Plus, medicine is up and coming and new things may be on the horizon. We have to stay positive and focused! How are you?

Danielle: Yes, we do! Never lose hope and always remain faithful. God has big things in store for all of us. So, you had your port put in? How was that? My actual port site didn't hurt but where they ran the wires up into my neck was super sore. I hope your treatments don't make you sick and if they do, they manage your medicine to help you. Are they giving you Zofran?

Alli: Yes, I have Zofran. My neck hurts from where they pulled or whatever they did when they put the port in. Just hoping it all stays clean and working so I don't have to face any other obstacles. But I'm ready to fight and so happy to have the support group I do. Thank you for all your help and answering questions for me.

I couldn't let these people down. I couldn't let my boyfriend down. I couldn't let my mom and dad down as they sat there looking at me as the chemo was pumped into my body.

During the treatment, I began to feel light-headed. My tongue felt thick and I was talking with a lisp. My dad knew what was happening. His eyes filled with tears knowing I was having a negative reaction to the drugs. He called immediately for the nurse to return. Soon, there were so many people in the room asking me questions, giving me more medicine, and reminding me that it was going to be okay. *Was it though? Was it okay that I was having a reaction to the chemo that was supposed to be killing the cancer?*

My dad posted on the Rally for Alli page that my first treatment was over, and it was rough. "Allison is now home with a 48-hour pump and resting." Andrew, Miranda, and the boys came up that weekend to see me. Eric came home and his parents came up to visit. They all hung out in the tiny living room and I slept on and off throughout the weekend. Sunday came when I could happily say goodbye to the pump and tearfully say goodbye to Eric and my visitors. Then the sickness started. Throwing up from the nausea made my brain hurt and left me with a feeling that I wanted to die.

ALLISON LIPPMAN, THIS IS YOUR REALITY

In the early weeks of July 2017, I had about eight days of nausea, diarrhea, vomiting, chills, sweating…name every disgusting symptom and I had it after the first chemo treatment. I was weak and incredibly sick. This was going to be my life every two weeks. I went to the main downtown Dallas hospital for my second treatment. This round, my mom and Eric's mom were with me. I slept through most of the treatment until I started to feel that sickening reaction again. I had to fight through it. I wanted every last drop of chemo to kill this cancer, but the charge nurse told me, "No, not this time." I was having the same allergic reaction and needed to stop the Oxaliplatin.

I was wheelchaired out of the hospital. Back at home, I settled in for the weekend with Polly Pocket, my nickname for the pump. The pump was programmed to infuse Fluorouracil (5FU) very slowly into my body. I should have called Polly Pocket something worse since I hated "her." I had a belt around my waist that held the pump. Over Friday and Saturday, every few minutes I could hear it disperse medicine into me. By Sunday afternoon, it would beep to let me know it was empty. Then the routine would begin again. I would call my mom into the room to disconnect me. She would pull the tape off my chest, pump saline, and tell me to hold my breath as she pulled the needle out of the port.

Like clockwork after this procedure, I would get sick. My mom, dad, and Eric became my constant caregivers; driving me wherever I needed to go, giving me precise medicine at the precise time, cooking, cleaning, doing laundry, cleaning out my throw-up bucket, drawing a bath, and generally caring for me. I was no longer a 31-year-old healthy woman, the general manager of a hotel, or a girlfriend who made dinner, cleaned, did laundry, and traveled with her super boyfriend. I was a cancer patient, a sick cancer patient. I recall my dad lying in bed with me, crying and asking, "Why do you have to be so sick? I just want to take this out of you and put it in me." "No!" I would always bark back, "I couldn't imagine watching you be as sick as me."

It was after my second treatment when I was running fingers through my hair and clumps started to fall out. My mom brought the trash can to me as I threw away handfuls of hair and cried my eyes out. This was the moment I dreaded. My mom suggested that maybe if I cut my hair short, it would be easier to manage. My mom, dad, and Eric went downstairs with me to the salon in the apartment complex. My mom briefed the hairdresser on my illness, who reassured me it would all be okay. I cried the entire time I was in the salon chair. I still cry when I hear "A Thousand Years" by Christina Perri, the song that was playing as she washed my hair and I could feel her pulling it out. Eric sat beside me and held my hand as tears rolled down during this dreaded event. She brushed and the handfuls of hair that came out were placed under the towels on her cart. I knew she was trying to hide it from me, but I could feel it. I could feel my scalp being exposed with every brush stroke that took my hair out. She began to chop it into a bob. I cried. I cried as she kept cutting it shorter and shorter. I finally said that was enough and was getting tired and needed to leave. She styled my hair. My parents and Eric told me how beautiful I looked; while all I could see was a pile of my hair under the towel with my gaunt face under this new chopped bob. I gave the hairdresser my credit card for the $35 cut. My dad quickly pushed aside my card and said he would pay for this haircut. Back in the apartment, I patted my head that was tender from all the hair that was pulled out.

SUMMER 2017, THE WORST OF TIMES, THE BEST OF TIMES

Earlier in July, Eric called Father Alfonse, our priest in Dallas, to ask if he would come to the apartment to give me the sacrament of anointing of the sick. I couldn't believe I was at the point of receiving this sacrament before marriage. It was not the order I wanted in my life. I cried throughout the sacrament but quickly found comfort with Father Alfonse. He helped me find a renewed purpose for my faith.

I always leaned heavily on my faith but never how it may impact my own mortality. I don't know how many Hail Mary's I said as I laid in bed every night, trying not to throw up, or every time I took a bite of food and prayed it would stay down. I knew God was present in the midst of this storm. The easy thing to do is to turn my back and dwell in self-pity. There were definitely times when I felt like this, but most of the time, I was thankful. I was thankful it wasn't me who had to watch my family or Eric throwing their guts up, bleeding from the rectum because of so many bowel movements, dry heaving because there was nothing in their stomach to soak up the medicine, pulling their hair or witnessing it fall out, or watching the scale drop 4-plus pounds every week.

Speaking of weight loss, I've always struggled with my weight. I've tried every fad diet there is. I'm obsessed with weight loss. At first, I was sitting comfortably in size 10 jeans. Soon, my jeans were slipping off my waist and I was downsizing to a 6. Then, size 6 was loose and I dropped to a size 2. I remember trying on my petite sister-in-law's jeans, and they fit. I cried. I cried because I knew I was extremely sick. In a normal dieting world, I would be happy. My uncle told me I was, "The perfect body for clothes." I know that statement came from love and compassion, but I think it made me go into a downward spiral. I looked like a Holocaust prisoner. I could see and count my ribs. I had lost so much weight that my skin was sagging. Eric would always tell me that I was still pretty, but my eyes were shallow and my face was gaunt. My body was exactly what you'd think of when someone says cancer. I was being eaten alive by this disease. I wasn't pretty. I couldn't do anything. I couldn't have sex anymore because it hurt, and Eric felt like he was going to hurt me. I'll never forget him telling me in bed one night that he was afraid he would snap me in half.

Night-time was the worst. I was alone. I would think. I was so drugged up throughout the day as I tried to function; moving from the bed to couch to bed. I barely ate despite everyone yelling at me to eat protein shakes, granola bars, fat-rich yogurt, anything. I remember going to McAllister's with Eric one day when I felt slightly better. I ordered a sandwich but immediately felt ill. We had to leave and I took my whole sandwich home with me. I worked at eating that stupid sandwich for a week. I nibbled a piece, then threw up, then looked at it and got so mad. I still can't go to McAllister's to this day. Every bad incident leaves a memory; such as the highway exit to the hospital where this whole journey started, Nordstrom's main floor where I threw up because I was overcome by the smell of too much perfume, particular gas stations where my mom would stop for my emergencies as she drove me from Dallas to Camp Creek, restaurants where I got sick from the sight and smell of a plate of food, and even gummies or lemon drop candies, which I thought I could stuff in my mouth non-stop...until I got sick and threw everything up in vivid orange and yellow vomit. Not a pretty picture to store in the memory bank.

The summer of 2017 felt like an eternity. I would be in Dallas for treatments but then go to the lake house with my parents while Eric was at work. I was helpless; couldn't drive, couldn't prepare food, couldn't find the strength to get up to get my own medicine. Miranda bought me a doorbell to ring so everyone in the other room could come help me when I needed a bucket to throw up in, pain medicine or an extra blanket. This dire situation was taking a toll on Eric. He would have to drive from Dallas to my parents' home to see me. We could never really be alone. When we were, I was in bed while he took care of the household chores. Washing dishes never sounded so great to me until I couldn't do it. I physically could not stand over the sink and wash a dish. I could not get my own ice water because ice was too cold to touch with my neuropathy. I was becoming angry at myself and Eric was becoming desperate.

Eric finished his training and started flying the MD88. I was very proud of him. He would be home taking care of me, go fly a jet, then drive to Camp Creek to be with me. All he wanted to do was be with me. Eric turned to the church to find strength. At times I was mad, but I think it was because I was jealous. I hadn't been to church for months at this point because I was so sick. I remember one time when Eric was home; he had just flown with a captain who had changed to a holistic, raw-foods diet with his wife when she had breast cancer. Eric was desperate to help me. He had read and believed in this diet. He wanted me to read the book and start eating raw foods with him. He wrote me a letter:

***

Allison, The Love of My Life,

I Love you. A lot. You know this. I want to start with a concise statement that is the most important thing to me. You mean the world to me and the thought of losing you in any way terrifies me.

I am writing this in an attempt to convey my thoughts and feelings in the most clear way. It's been a while since we wrote emails to each other but I believe it works in conjunction with oral communications.

We've talked about this book briefly over the phone as I describe some things about the Hallelujah Diet; but as I leave it with you, I would like you to read it with an open mind and open heart. The things I've said about it are the most drastic changes in life. They are the things that caught my eye. I haven't properly or fully explained any of the reasons and logic behind the bold statements. In this I have faulted. I believe you'll quickly read and be able to understand the meaning behind the diet.

I believe in this diet. I know why but I can't fully explain through words what just reading about it and the hope it has given me has done to me. Many things happen for a reason in life. Somehow, right when you and I were both looking to put something other than career at the forefront of our lives, we found each other. It was an instantaneous and forever enduring bond. I believe there is a reason I was paired up to fly with Wade and open up about my situation. Wade was there to show us a path forward. There're many pilots who will sympathize with us, but Wade gave us a path forward to healing. I believe in my heart there was some divine intervention.

Since June when our lives took a dramatic turn overnight, we, our family, friends, and people we don't even know have offered prayers on our behalf. I have this calming feeling that this is one of the answers to those prayers. There may be other answers along the way as well but the Lord is giving us guidance. When I left for work last week, I was a wreck. I was scared about dropping one of the three therapy drugs and what this would do. I am scared to lose you. I love you. This may sound selfish but I would love another 60 or 70 years with you. Every day and moment we get to spend together going through this life as a team, I cherish. After reading this book over the last week, I've had a calming feeling throughout my body. Something unexplainable feels right.

I have changed since we started dating. It's all been for the better. Not one thing has been negative. I am definitely a more Christian and specifically Catholic Man. I have reprioritized my life without consciously thinking about it. It has just happened. This will be another big change in life. Switching almost everything we eat to something more wholesome and fresh will require some thought. Love, for your health and the ability to keep you here on Earth with me for another 60 years, I would do absolutely anything. We are in this together forever.

As you read the book, I hope we will be able to discuss while I'm at work and when I come home. If this is the lifestyle that we choose to take up, I pray and believe our families will support our decision. It may take a change of mentality regarding nutrition for many but the outcome will be worth all sacrifices. I have a strong conviction and deep burning heart feeling about this. That is something I still may not have been able to convey in words to you but I have no other way than to continue to share this diet and do it with you.

As you read this book, I am here. I pray you'll discuss it with me and keep an open mind and heart about what it takes, the sacrifices we'll give up, the new beautiful and delicious foods we'll try, and the vibrant renewed life and outlook that will be our reward. You

*and your family mean the world to me. You are the greatest person
I have come across in life and look forward to this new adventure
and many more to come in life.*

I love you with all my Heart,
Eric

***

How was I supposed to respond to this heartfelt plea? I was so lost. So desperate. So confused. So reluctant to adopt this diet because I just wanted to eat, no matter what I could get to stay down. It was the first time since this whole crisis started that made me question everything. Even to question Eric.

I talked to my parents about the diet and how much Eric believed in it. My dad told me that Eric desperately wanted to help and this was one way of reaching for a hopeful solution. As a father, he offered to talk to Eric. This terrified me, but I had no strength to battle it. *Great, now my dad has to talk to my boyfriend.* Eric was already stretched making those drives to the lake house where, like teenagers, we have supervised visits. I thought this talk with my dad would be the last straw to break his back and he will leave me. The talk went better than expected.

Unbeknown to me, when we went to the lake for July 4th, Eric asked my dad for my hand in marriage while they were sitting on the dock. They were closer than I ever realized.

Every two weeks in late July and early August the routine continued. Chemo was every fourteen days and I was sick thirteen of them. Not just morning sickness, but all-day sickness. I was wearing a nausea patch, popping medicine every few hours, and writing it down in my logbook so I didn't cross-dose myself with any of the fifteen prescriptions. Some days I was so sick, I had to stay in bed all day. It was a good day if I ate half a granola bar. I would ring my bedside bell for someone, anyone, to bring me medicine when the pain struck. I remember one day when I was so sick, I couldn't find the bell and literally cried, "Someone come help me."

FIRST COMES LOVE THEN COMES MARRIAGE

By mid-August, I was feeling weak but strong enough to venture out with Eric and my mom for the afternoon. It was always the three of us. Eric and I thought we might need a two-bedroom apartment so my mom could move in with us while she cared for me. Eric took us to lunch at a small Greek restaurant. I actually ate. I remember being so proud of myself for eating half of my gyro. Afterwards, my mom and I planned to get our nails done. Even though I was fading away, my hair was falling out, and death was advancing quicker than I would have hoped, it was still important to get my nails done.

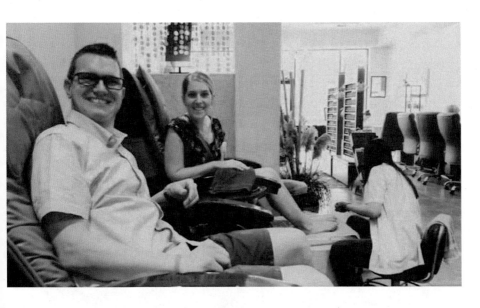

Eric came with us and even got a pedicure. He picked out a neutral pink color for me. I loved the color that Eric selected. I told him to remember the color because that will be what I want when we get engaged. I was (sort of) joking. I will remember the color C19 for the rest of my life.

August 17, 2017 - This was the day before my next chemo treatment and day thirteen since the last treatment, and I was feeling slightly better. I awoke, threw up, looked at Eric and asked, "Are you going to marry me?" That was my little attempt at humor when I was feeling so pathetic. Eric told me that he had a day-trip planned for us. We would try to do something on day twelve or thirteen because there would usually be a window of opportunity when I felt good enough to go for a cup of coffee or explore a new store in Dallas.

I didn't know where we were going, but Eric had the car packed, brought my medicine, a pillow, and my emergency bag. I decided to wear the blue and red dress that my dad bought me for my second date with Eric. As we drove along Highway 30 heading north of Dallas, we passed through Rockwall, Fate, Greenville, Campbell, Commerce, and then I saw a road sign that said *Paris 58 miles*. "Are we going to Paris?" I asked. "You'll see!" said Eric, piloting along without a signal of what was to be expected.

Paris, Texas, was the destination. We pulled up in the rain-soaked parking lot. I sensed that Eric had planned to recreate our joyful holiday in France from only a few months earlier. In the park is a replica of the Eiffel Tower that, unlike the Paris original, sports a giant-size, red cowboy hat. I was feeling that tourist vibe and took pictures as we walked toward the tower and Eric laid a blanket down. A French picnic was such a special idea for our day away. Like in France, we brought a tripod to pose for selfies. Before we sat down on the blanket, Eric said, "Let's go take a picture in

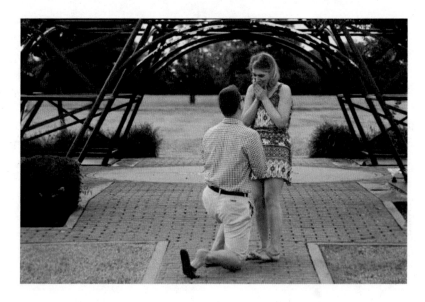

front of the tower." Nothing seemed out of the ordinary for Eric. Until he grabbed my hand in a way that he had never grabbed my hand before.

I could feel my armpits getting warm, feel my hands getting clammy, and feel my heartbeat in my throat. "Allison Claire Lippman, I love you." I am pretty sure that he said something about how much he loved traveling with me, how we go to church together, how we love each other's families, and "I can't imagine my life without you." He got down on one knee, opened a box to reveal a beautiful solitaire diamond ring, "Will you marry me?"

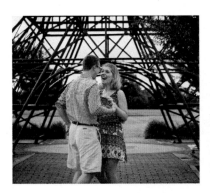 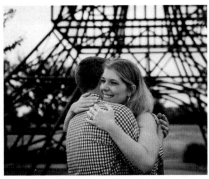

I had been on cloud nine when Eric first said, "I love you!" I was on cloud nine again, plus standing below the Eiffel Tower with mi amore. I hugged my man. I kissed him. He slid the ring onto my bony finger. That day, my hand looked so tiny and frail. But my nails looked fabulous. So did the ring. I looked over Eric's shoulder and saw his friend, Jamie, taking pictures. Eric had fulfilled all of my proposal requests: (1) ask my father for my hand, (2) make sure my nails are manicured and painted ahead of time, (3) use my full name when asking to marry me, (4) bend on one knee, and (5) hire a photographer to capture the raw emotions. Returning to the blanket under the behatted Eiffel Tower, Eric opened a bottle of champagne and handed me a box of macarons that he had a flight attendant bring back from France. My cunning fiancé thought of every last detail.

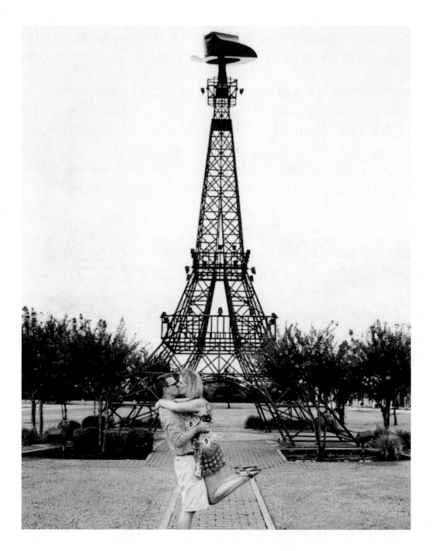

What I had not requested for the proposal must-haves was an audience. Lurking in a small building near the tower, our moms huddled to watch the whole proposal unfurl. They were aware of the surprise. There was no reason for us to call the mothers to announce the big news.

The ring was such a surprise. Eric and I had gone to look at engagement rings several months earlier. I was very particular about what I liked. Eric was even more particular in his questions about the ring to be sure he got every detail correct. Details I would not have known to ask about, but that's how Eric is. After I got sick, I didn't bring up the ring because I assumed an engagement and marriage would never happen. *Why would Eric spend money on a ring? What was he seeing in his future as my future was dwindling away?* Future wasn't a word in my current vocabulary. I concentrated my energy and hopes on one day at a time. But, on August 17, 2017, the possibility of a future with Eric blazed into my confused brain.

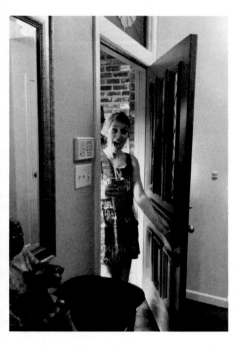

After Paris and the surprise of a lifetime, we returned home for a much-needed nap. I should have been exhausted but my adrenaline kept me going. We had previously arranged to go to my aunts Marilyn and Mary Ann's house for dinner with my parents that evening. When we pulled up, my dad greeted us in the driveway. He grabbed my hand and hugged me. I was excited to see him. I knew he was in town to go with me to chemo the next day. But when I opened the front door to the house, I was shocked by a room full of...everyone!

Everyone, who had been invited by Eric to come celebrate, had been told he was going to propose to me. Andrew, Miranda, Jack, and baby Ben snuck in from Tomball. My Uncle Sheldon flew in from Austin. All of our parents, brothers, aunts, uncles, and cousins were in from all over Texas. I was overwhelmed that everyone had traveled to be with us. They had truly swept me off my feet. The dining room was decorated, food was plentifully spread across the table, and so much love was in the air. I was feeling better than I had in weeks. Eric and I spent the evening chatting with family, taking pictures, and showing off the hell-of-a-rock on my hand.

Miranda made a t-shirt that read, *Pop the Champagne, I'm Changing my Last Name!*

Eric had thought out every detail so precisely. It was a magical day. I felt incredibly loved. These folks who filled the room were my future. I had to

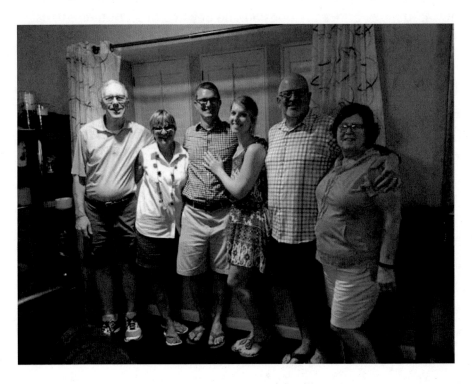

fight for them. I had to fight for Eric. I was feeling so great that I thought I should skip chemo that week, but that did not happen. I wore the t-shirt to chemo the next day and showed off my ring.

The post for Rally for Alli that day said, "Alli is headed into round 5 with a little more weight on her left hand." I couldn't wait to show my nurses on Friday morning. I walked in proudly with my shirt and held out my hand. They would jokingly back up when I flashed my ring as it was rather large, especially on my twig-thin fingers.

Days and weeks went by. I tried to start planning my dream wedding on days I was feeling better. Those days were starting to become fewer and fewer. My appointments at the oncologist were not very hopeful. I enjoyed seeing Dr. Beg and his wonderful nurses, my friend Jaime, and being together with my family. However, I was always hearing that the tumors were "stable." As my dad said, in the cancer world, stable is good. It also meant the tumors were not shrinking. It meant I would keep doing chemo.

As September 2017 approached, my hair continued to fall out to the point where a slouchy beanie was the source of comfort to cover my balding

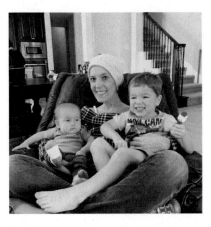

head. It was also during this time, that I was choosing the venue for our wedding reception and trying to make big decisions and big plans for our upcoming nuptials. I always wanted a fall wedding but with my declining health putting pressure on our timeline, we selected April 28, 2018, as our wedding date.

I went to Tomball to spend a few days with Andrew, Miranda, Jack and Ben at the end of October. It was hard to be in a different home and feel so ill. I wanted to hold Ben and play with Jack. I was so weak that I could hardly pick Jack up without a real struggle. I remember sitting on the couch and holding Ben when suddenly the nausea hit and I had to launch him into Miranda's arms so I could run to the bathroom and throw up. My little Jack would try to tug at my cap and I would tell him "No" so he wouldn't get frightened by my bald head and skeleton-like body.

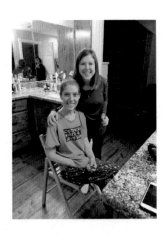
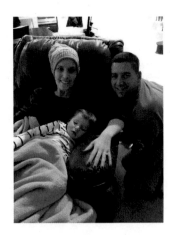

GETTING WIGGY IN A WIG

Miranda took me to a small wig shop. The time had come that I needed to cover my head with a wig. I tried a short brown wig. Eric had never seen me with brown hair, but we all liked it. It brought out my green eyes. However, the lady told us that a new shipment would come later that afternoon, so we returned home and waited for her to call us. Usually I waited for a hair trim or a color appointment, but never to get a wig. I felt so weird but ready to have a normal haircut. I had to embrace the fear of losing my hair.

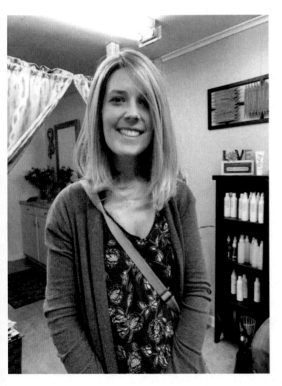

We went back to the wig shop where I tried on a blondish brown wig. It was me. My hair looked exactly like it did before I got sick. Miranda took pictures of me so we could see how it looked photographically. Jack said he liked it. Eric's smile was as big as it was the day I said yes to marrying him. I went outside to see how it looked in the natural sunlight. When I went back into the shop to pay, Eric handed me a bag with my special shampoo, conditioner, and wig stand. He and his parents bought my wig and made me the happiest girl, again.

I had my wig and felt somewhat normal when I wore it. I was self-conscious because I still looked like a cancer patient as I withered away under my wig. I would never let Eric see me put my wig on or take it off. I would shut the door and put my beanie on so that my bald head was never exposed. I slept in my beanie, I took a bath with my beanie, and if I ever needed to take it off to wash my head, I would close the bathroom door. However, one day being so sick, I laid in bed all day. *Is this really who Eric wants to marry?* He laid with me and I slowly took off my beanie. My heart was beating fast. I was nervous but determined that he had to see me, the person to whom he was committing his life. He cried and told me I was beautiful. I was disgusted but overcome with so much love for Eric at the same time. I had to commit to him.

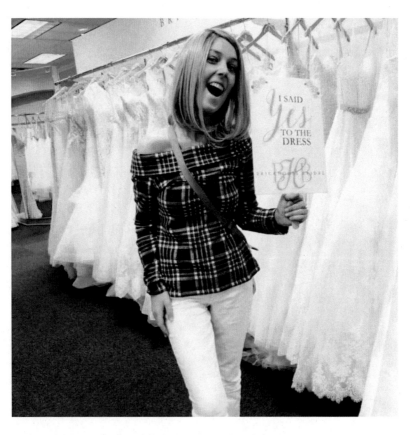

Miranda invited me to Houston between chemo weeks to look for wedding dresses with her and my mom. I never thought the day would come. There I was clipping pink tags on the dresses that I liked. I went to the dressing room and started to undress. I was wearing a small bralette and saggy underwear. I slipped into a dress that was gorgeous but consumed my frail body. I looked like a little girl playing dress up in my mom's closet. I flashed on a memory from high school when my friend Sky and I went to a *quinceañera* dress shop in the mall. We filled the dressing rooms up with these huge, elaborate dresses and tried them on. The little sales-lady yelled at us for not hanging them up properly.

Play time was over now. I had a dress consultant with me. She helped me get in the dress. As I repositioned my wig, I told her my story. I told her that I used to be a size 10 and now I don't even think a 0 fits me. She clamped the dress tighter so I could see the form of it on my body. It was beautiful.

I walked out of the dressing room and saw Miranda and my mom's face light up. For a while, I didn't feel like a cancer patient. I felt like a bride-to-be getting ready to marry the kindest man in the world. I tried on two other dresses just to compare. Feeling weak from the changing, I knew that I couldn't find anything I loved more than the first dress. My mom proudly paid for my dress. I think, in this instance, hope overcame her.

At this point, I had completed ten rounds of Folfirinox chemotherapy. I was experiencing a side effect of neuropathy. My body continued to wither away. The doctors feared permanent damage if I continued with additional rounds. Most patients can only stand ten to twelve rounds and he was satisfied that I was able to "tolerate" the ten rounds. He said I would start to feel better without the strongest chemo drug.

Into November, I was excited for this change from the chemo regimen and a possibility of feeling better and easing myself back to work part-time. We all had hope at that point that I would be able to eat and start living a more normal life. I was still taking morphine and other medicines so I would not be able to drive myself to work.

When the morning came for me to go back to the hotel, I was crippled with fear. I used to be so confident in my career, but all that confidence had disappeared that day. I had to dress and put on my wig to look presentable as a working woman. As I dressed, I cried so hard I couldn't breathe. Eric heard me and came in and held me.

As he drove me to work, I could feel my heart beating in my throat. He dropped me off around 10 AM which is usually when I would be waking up to begin my day at home in sick mode. I didn't do much work that first day back. In fact, the temporary manager who was filling in for me had arranged for a staff lunch so I could see everyone. It was a bit awkward to walk into my office and have someone else sitting in my chair and doing my job. I was thankful he was there. I didn't want to step on his toes and he didn't want to step on mine. I think it was understood that coming to work, even for a couple hours a day, helped me feel a bit more normal and help divert attention from my illness. I wasn't much help, but the manager told me it was motivating for the staff to see me. We were family and I understood what that meant. As soon as I saw everyone's face, I felt more at ease.

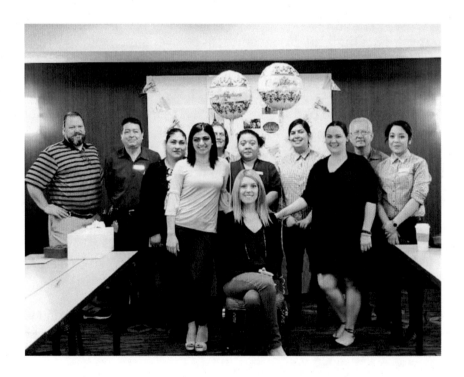

Despite the welcoming morning back in the office, I called Eric around 1 PM to pick me up as I was completely exhausted. Three hours of sitting and talking was enough to make me want to go home and sleep the rest of the evening. I was disappointed in myself for not being able to stay at the hotel longer and trying to do some actual work. In my prime, a ten to twelve-hour day was normal. Now, after three hours of chit-chatting, I was done.

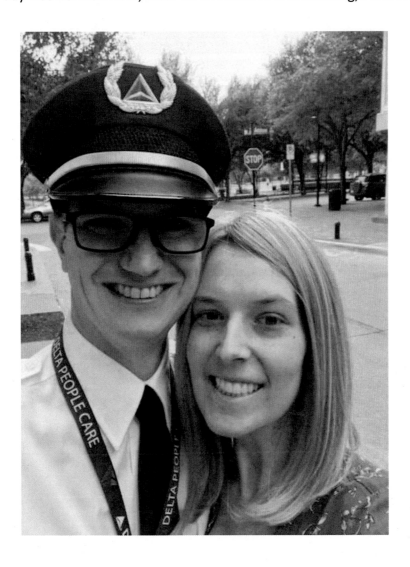

I was also embarrassed and felt like a sympathy case. I could only do this routine for two or three days a week, usually toward the end of the two-week mark before I went back for chemo. Eric or my mom would have to drive me to work. I was never left alone.

After chemo, I was out for a week battling the same symptoms. They didn't seem to ease up after the last drug was taken out of the cocktail. I would tell the hotel staff to expect me at 10 AM. By 11, I would text them to say it wasn't happening that day. I was the worst employee. I adored my boss and it was defeating to feel like I was letting him down. He was my "Uncle Mike." He sent me the blanket that I took to every chemo appointment. He was the reason I wanted to get back to work.

At the same time as I was trying to go back to work, Eric and I began marriage prep classes at church. We went to the sponsor-couple's house for an evening, every few weeks. The meetings were a bit awkward to attend as the conversations to ensure we were compatible seemed silly. *Like if we have agreed to get married, don't you think we would have already discussed some of these things? To go over all of them again with a couple that we barely know is just a bit...forced.* I remember one evening when the sponsor asked if we were rushing to get married because of "the cancer." It was like a slap in the face but also kind of made me question what Eric saw for his future.

We went home after that meeting and I cried asking Eric why he wanted to marry me. *Won't it be less painful to just take the ring back now and save our money and not go through all this and just enjoy the final days together?* He cried uncontrollably, to where I had to console him and remind him to breathe. He just kept saying, "I can't lose you. I can't lose you." Looking back, all those questions we had to answer in the counseling were silly compared to that moment when we both knew we completed each other. We physically couldn't live without each other. I had to fight with any strength left in my body to make it to that wedding on April 28.

ALL I WANT FOR CHRISTMAS IS YOU & ME

Christmas 2017 was approaching. It seemed like ten years had passed since I was diagnosed in June. A few days before Christmas, I was supposed to go to dinner with my aunts, Marilyn and Mary Ann, and uncles, Sheldon and John, who had come to visit me at my apartment in Addison. We had reservations at the Italian restaurant below my apartment. By dinnertime, they had to go without me because my pain was crippling. When I went to the bathroom to try and find relief from the pain, I was shocked to see the toilet filled with blood unlike I had ever seen before. It felt like my stomach was full of nails as I cried and screamed in pain. I called my dad, who called my should-have-been dinner companions at the restaurant and told them to hurry back to the apartment. When things had calmed down, I was able to visit with my aunts and uncles who sat at the foot of my bed chatting to take my mind off of the pain. I had a rough night. My aunts stayed with me while I waited for mom to drive from Camp Creek to Dallas in the early morning hours. I had become dependent on having my parents with me. I was anxious without them.

Driving to Dallas was the norm for my mom. When she arrived, we went immediately to the ER where I was given Diprivan to help ease the pain and let me finally rest. After being released from the ER, I was able to go to Houston with my mom to celebrate Christmas with the family.

Christmas Eve has always been a day of love and fun for my family. Andrew and my dad usually go play pool and we all celebrate in the evening after Mass. Christmas Mass has always been my favorite. I love to dress up and see everyone get ready for their festivities. It's like the final moment of the hustle and bustle and something you always see in the movies. Then we come home and eat the yummiest snacks like Scotch eggs, tamales, and drink a few too many bottles of wine between all of us. I know this isn't the norm for most families, but we have always been close and enjoy creating a joyous mood in the house. Christmas Eve has always been one of my favorite evenings of the year.

This year was different. I wasn't allowed to go to Mass because of the germs that I may catch. I remember crying on the couch because I wasn't allowed to go. I wanted to have a normal Christmas Eve if it was to be my last. Andrew offered to stay. My mom offered. My dad, too. No one wanted me to be alone, but I wanted everyone to be together. It was just fueling the fire. My sweet three-year-old nephew, Jack, walked over to me and held my arm. I didn't think he understood what was going on but, oh, he did. He knew I was sad, scared, and not ready to say my last Merry Christmas. My mom ended up staying with me as the others went to Mass while I napped on the couch.

When they came home, we all sat on the couch together as I continued to nap on and off. Everyone had plates of food but I couldn't even stand the thought of tasting a small cracker. I usually had to force myself to drink a protein shake or Ensure to get calories in me, but I often threw it up and afterwards couldn't get the powdery chocolate taste out of my mouth. The only taste I could manage was the flavor of the pot gummies that my aunt bought me.

As we watched TV and enjoyed the fire, I suddenly felt hands on my forehead as someone leaned in to kiss me. It was my pilot. My Eric. Eric had a very short layover from his schedule and took the time to come to Houston to surprise me. This was a love-fueled, life-altering moment. On this Christmas Eve, it was like a heavenly angel reached down and touched me to tell me it wasn't my turn yet. Heaven can wait. Eric was my angel telling me not to give up.

The last two weeks of any year always seem like a blur with the excitement of Christmas and New Years and the abundance of food, drinks, parties, and friends and family coming and going. Sadly, or perhaps fortunately, I could vaguely remember the months before this whole episode with the diagnosis, the chemo, the pain, and the loss of hair. Without the photos and video to look at, I could barely remember the details of the trip to France with Eric in the spring. My life was a blur.

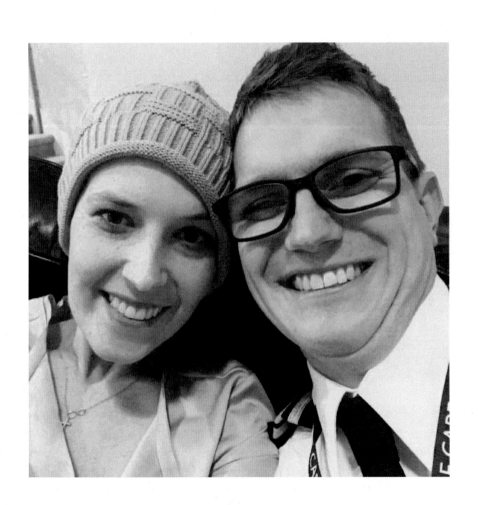

After what turned out to be my last chemo treatment on December 29 and the drugs had worn off, I told my mom that I was done with chemo. *How long could I live without this poison that was sickening me and threatening whatever quality of life was left for me and Eric?*

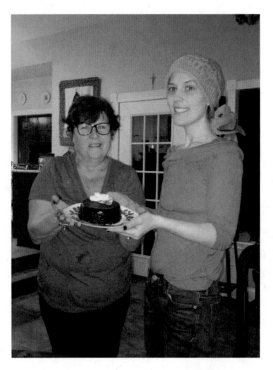

At a previous December staging appointment just a few weeks prior to this final chemo treatment, Dr. Beg mentioned additional spots were found in surrounding lymph nodes and recommended we look at potential alternative treatments. We had no idea what those alternatives might be, but Dr. Beg had set the wheels turning toward a possibility earlier in my diagnosis.

When I was first diagnosed, Dr. Beg was perplexed why I, as a young woman, had this form of cancer. He suggested that we do genetic profiling of my tumor. The procedure was done and Dr. Beg sent the biopsy of my tumor to First Health Solutions in Boston, that specialize in genomics. Dr. Beg told us that 99% of results usually come back negative. This did not seem like a hopeful situation, but there is always that 1% potential for positive news. Weeks after the biopsy had been sent, Dr. Beg had a surprise from First Health Solutions. "Boston called. And they never call." The researchers found a mutation called RET fusion and felt it could be a gateway for a future trial. This was the good news, but I still had to run the course of conventional chemo. Dr. Beg was hesitant to stop chemotherapy until it was clearly no longer working. This news came in August. Chemo treatments continued for another four months.

On December 31, 2017, my mom pulled out the needle from my port for the last time.

The search began for an alternative treatment since I had made the decision not to continue with chemo. My mom contacted MD Anderson to see if I qualify for a trial that targets my specific mutation, RET fusion. The appointment was made and I waited for my next adventure to start.

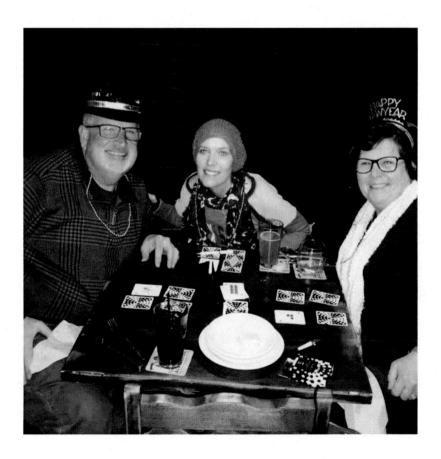

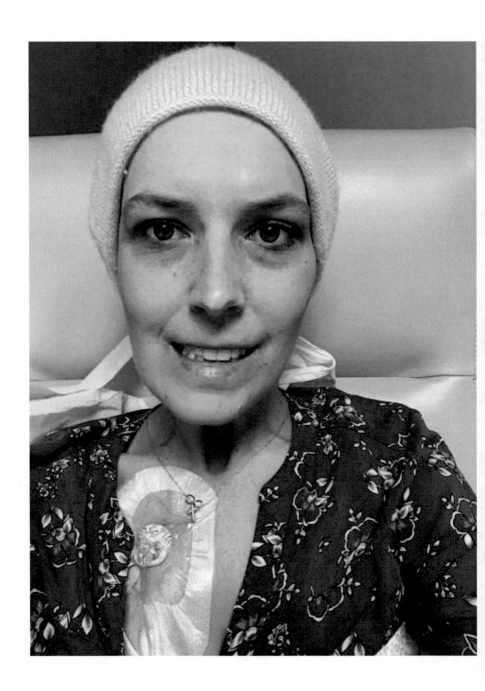

WITH THE NEW YEAR COMES NEW HOPE

January 2018 – Eric and I spent the first weekend of January celebrating Cathy's 65th birthday in San Antonio. I used every drop of energy to share in the celebration but spent a lot of time in the hotel bed.

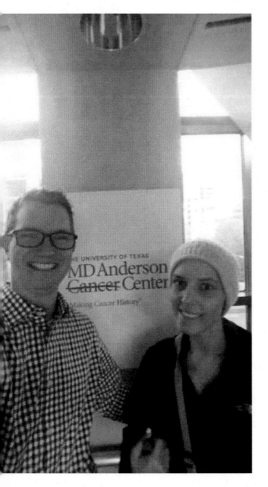

My parents joined Eric and me in Houston for an appointment on January 8. We all got hotel rooms in the Houston Medical Center. All of us were having a restless night. My dad knocked on my door to ask for a Restoril (a sleeping pill). I think our nerves were getting the best of us. I gave him a handful of my pills.

We went to MD Anderson the next day. Eric stopped me to take a picture in front of the MD Anderson sign. I said, "Why are we doing this?" He said it was a new beginning. I reluctantly posed. Eric sent it to my family and Miranda posted it on the Rally for Alli site. That picture represents a monumental moment in my life. I am glad Eric thought to document it.

I met with Dr. Subbiah, who was excited to start a new trial with my very specific mutation. Dr. Subbiah is in charge of the trial I qualified for and has a larger-than-life personality. You can hear him coming down the hallway as he enthusiastically meets each of his patients. He told me I needed to stop chemo immediately and start this trial at MD Anderson.

They were on the horizon with a new trial that targets RET fusion. As he filled my head with information, he looked me in the eye and enthusiastically asked, "When is your wedding?" I responded, "Um, April 28." His reply, "You'll have hair by then."

The vibrant doctor quickly retreated to the back of the room when Dr. Javle, the head of the GI department at MD Anderson, entered. He learned of my case when he met Dr. Kuban, my future father-in-law, at a seminar in Dallas earlier that fall. David showed my records to Dr. Javle who encouraged us to call MD Anderson. As fate would have it, I was shaking his hand that morning. Dr. Subbiah seemed surprised that I was already known by his colleagues at MD Anderson.

I met with the trial coordinator, Anna, who was a young lady with a lab coat pocket lined with multi-colored ballpoint pens. I sat with Anna as she reviewed packets of information to explain what the protocols and regulations were as I started a new medicine. I had to sign off in agreement to each page as I quickly learned what would be required of me. I had to document the exact time I took the medicine and be sure my meals did not interfere. I had to wait two hours before I took the medicine and one hour after. I also had to stay away from grapefruit juice as it could inhibit the success of the medicine.

As much hope as the trial presented, there was also a significant downside that I learned as I read through the instructions. Pregnancy was prohibited as researchers did not know how this medicine would affect me, much less a baby. I also feared the long-term effects that the last six months of poisonous chemotherapy might have on a fetus. A permanent birth control was required.

A MIRACLE IN BLUE PILLS

January 24, 2018 - The first day of the LOXO-292 trial consisted of several blood draws and labs to research how the new medicine would affect my body. I went from a 48-hour "Polly Pocket" pump with its toxic medicines to taking four blue pills per day. I swallowed two pills in the morning and two in the evening. I still had other pills to manage the residual side effects from chemotherapy.

Within days, those previous symptoms were slowly dwindling away. I began weaning myself off morphine but increasing the Xanax to control my anxiety. I was anxious because of the unknown on this new trial. I was also becoming more aware of how sick I really was for the last few months. I was coming out of the fog from all my medicines and realizing the world that surrounded me.

Feeling better, I was able to go back to the hotel and work more hours as my energy increased. There were new staff members at the hotel who had not known me before I became sick. Some people did not know my previous work ethic and the time I spent to earn my position. One new person could not understand why old friends were speaking so highly of me; she was not impressed with my return. Her comments were a slap in the face that would change my outlook on my return to the job that I loved and worked hard to get.

YIN MEETS YANG

During February and March 2018, the new LOXO protocol regimen required frequent trips from Dallas to MD Anderson. Someone, either my parents or Eric, had to drive me and be with me at these appointments and observations. The observations were required to monitor how I reacted to the new medicines, requiring eight hours in a hospital bed. This was a time for the doctors to acquire research data for the drug's use on a pancreatic cancer patient. They monitored my vitals, frequently drew blood, and performed EKGs every two hours.

During these long hours in a hospital bed and being observed, I kept busy on my laptop as I escaped one unknown reality and retreated to the more hopeful planning of a perfect wedding. I had my dream wedding planned in my head for years and was working to bring it to life. I had all of my favorite chick flicks in my repertoire of details that would help me to create the most epic day. Most importantly, I could check off having a perfect groom.

As I shared my dreams with Eric, he began researching the details. Eric has a keen eye for details. In fact, this was one of the qualities I loved about him. He could take my big dream and find a workable plan. As he would research the small details of my big picture, he added his opinions - *oops!* - which I did not always want to hear. *There would be no interference with my dream.* As an example, for the reception, Eric wanted us to buy everything for the bar: the lemons, limes, mixers, sodas, beers, wine, liquor, and only have the catering company serve. I wanted to have the catering company bring everything, set up the bar, and serve the drinks at the reception. His plan completely overwhelmed me. I couldn't wrap my head around dealing with the small details as opposed to simply hiring the company to manage that part of the reception. Compromising was an early lesson Eric and I learned. Eric had compromised enough by just being with me. I wanted my dream wedding, but I also wanted my dream groom to be happy.

At this same time, I was informed that the hotel where I worked in Dallas was being sold and a new management company was being considered. Changing companies in the midst of the changes that I was already enduring was daunting. It felt like that metaphorical straw that would break the camel's back. I worked remotely from the hospital to ensure I was a good candidate for the job as general manager with the new company.

When I returned to Dallas from one of the MD Anderson trips, I had to schedule the first of many interviews for general manager; the job that I already had with the current management company. Still feeling sick and weak, I had to "dress for success." I found clothes that fit my still thin frame, adjusted my wig to look natural, took a Xanax for my nerves, and repeated the mantra "one exit at a time."

Ironically, I had to take a break from my desk as the general manager to drive across Dallas to interview with the new management company. It was with the general manager of another hotel in their portfolio. Max was pompous and did not impress me, but I was there to impress him. He had an arrogance that reminded me of the original oncologist who had an impersonal bedside manner. This type of arrogance does not work in the hospitality industry either. Max asked how my leave of absence affected my team. I explained my diagnosis and determination to get back to the job that I have been successful at. After my explanation, he looked at the diamond ring on my left hand, leaned back in his office chair and scoffed, "When is the big day?" and "Do you really want to do that?" If looks could kill, then my expression to Max was: *Don't question the one good thing in my life.*

After a string of interviews, I did get the job.

Returning to a 10 to 12-hour work day, I toiled my ass off. I no longer had the tenure earned with the previous management company. There was quite a bit of staff turnover during my leave of absence. I was trying to build confidence with the new employees who were skeptical of me and this new management company. The stress of the job and the uncertainty of the new medical trial left me exhausted.

I was regularly meeting Kelly, the wedding planner, in College Station. As I wanted to put the finishing touches on décor, menus, and playlists, she knew my reality. Kelly suggested we arrange for a cot to be in my dressing room for any needed naps or rests on our big day. At the time, this sounded like a much-needed detail that I never wanted to include in my plans.

Wedding bells were the prelude to my new reality as a married woman. I was in the final countdown to becoming Mrs. Kuban. I meticulously created a spreadsheet of details for the wedding, as well as a daily checklist for staff during the ten days that I would be away from the hotel; the most auspicious and magical week of my life!

HERE COMES THE BRIDE AND GROOM

As I walked out the sliding doors of the hotel on April 24, 2018, I thought of how many times I had walked in and out of that place as a changed person: leaving for my 30th birthday trip, going on a first date with Eric, leaving for France with Eric as my beau, enduring crippling pain, rushing to the emergency room and receiving my cancer diagnosis, returning to the job with a wig, being hired by a new management team, and soon to be returning as a married woman. Eric arrived as my dashing prince; not on a white horse but in his trusty Nissan Xterra, that I lovingly call Nancy.

Eric and I headed south on Interstate 45 toward College Station to embark on the greatest adventure of our lives. We arrived at my parent's home at Camp Creek that evening to get the weekend started. My dad and I practiced the father-daughter dance in the living room. Tears filled my eyes as we moved across the floor to a true Texas love song, **From Here to the Moon and Back** by Willie Nelson and Dolly Parton. "Love everlasting, I promise you that." With one twirl under my dad's arm, my wig wiggled. That near disaster prompted a note on my wedding spreadsheet: extra hairpins to keep my wig in place.

Eric and I also practiced our first dance in the large living room of my parent's home. This practice space was a far cry from the patch of available floor space in our small apartment in Addison. Eric and I also had selected the ideal song for our first dance. Each word of Ed Sheeran's **Perfect** was accurate about our relationship. "So in love fighting against all odds." There was also a line, "To carry love, to carry children of our own" that was gut-wrenching for us, a couple about to take vows as husband and wife and having been told that getting pregnant was out of the question while on the clinical trial.

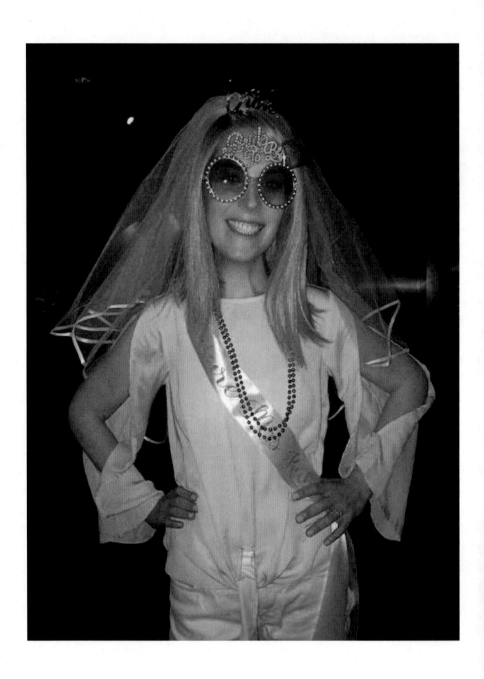

APRIL 28, 2018!

Perhaps it was the magic of the day finally arriving or the new chemicals circulating through my body, but the wedding seems to have flown by, somewhat a blur in my memory. Yet, there are specific moments that are ingrained in my heart.

As my bridesmaids and I settled into the bridal suite, two of Eric's groomsmen came in with special gifts. Each of the bridesmaids received their individual favorite Starbucks coffee order that Eric had collected from them earlier. I was handed a huge box with many individually wrapped boxes inside and a card that instructed me to open one gift each hour as I got ready.

All the girls' and my hair were pinned into gorgeous curls. Fake eyelashes completed the perfect face make-up. Finally slipping into my gown, I looked into the full-length mirror for the first time fully dressed and coiffed. I felt so beautiful. My makeup was flawless. The fake eyelashes accentuated my green eyes. My wig was styled in a beautiful updo. I looked like a real bride and was ready to marry Eric and live a normal life.

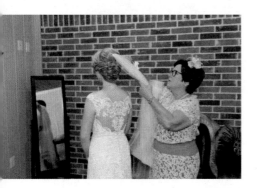

My mom came into the bridal suite to see me before the wedding ceremony. She gasped and held her hand over her heart. She had been skeptical of the wedding plans early in my diagnosis, but all that skepticism

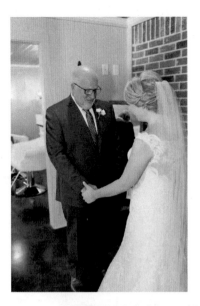

vanished from her face as she looked in awe at a healthy and beautiful bride in front of her.

As a surprise for my dad, I had the label changed inside of the suit that he ordered for the wedding. Instead of reading "This suit is for Phil Lippman," it read "This suit is for My Little Girl." He said he cried when he got it and was sure they would be the first of many happy tears to come.

I dreamed of the moment when my dad would first see me in my wedding dress.

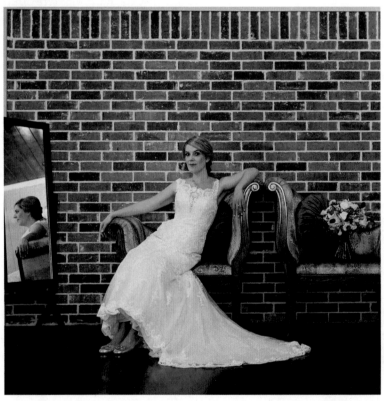

That dream came true. He walked into the bridal suite and hugged me. I felt a wet tear on my cheek. He looked at me and blubbered, "I knew this was going to happen." I cried as well. These tears were shed for the pain and the uncertainty of the past months and for the hopefulness of this moment and the future.

Before leaving for the church, the bridesmaids and I took pictures outside by the lake. I was overcome with heat and dizziness, much like I felt when going through chemo. Maybe it was nerves. Maybe it was excitement.

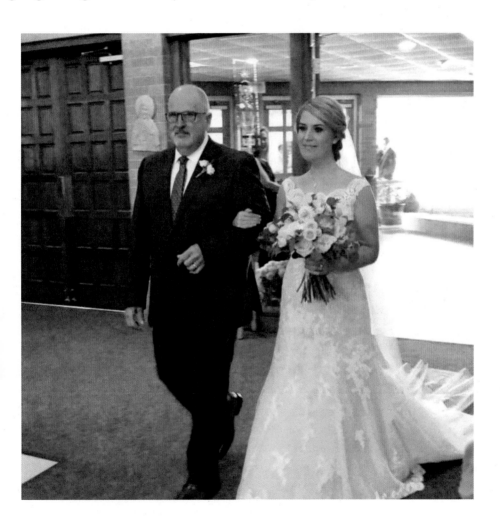

Maybe it was the chemicals in my body. *Why is it happening on this of all days?* I had some relief when we got into the limo heading to St. Thomas Aquinas Church and felt the blast of air conditioning. In the church, I sat down in the back room and closed my eyes as we waited.

The ceremony began. The bridesmaids walked down the aisle as the soloist sang **Set Me as a Seal**. The doors to the sanctuary were closed, giving my dad and me one last private moment. My time had come. As we walked down the aisle, I saw the faces and looked in the eyes of family and friends who had traveled from Europe and across the States. The excitement of finally seeing each other after the last several months was a cherished moment. Somehow, I mustered the strength and calmness to walk joyously down the aisle. It was finally time to share in a happy moment together and not share health updates.

I looked toward Eric as my dad and I inched closer to him. He looked so handsome in his three-piece suit with a smile on his face that broadly reached both ears. I could see the nervous laughter he always has when he stands still and smiles for a picture. My dad hugged his little girl for the final time as Miss Lippman before placing my hand in Eric's. As my dad released from our hug, his suit sleeve caught my veil that came unpinned from my wig and fell to the ground. *Thank God it was the veil and not the whole damn wig.*

Eric and I asked Father Alfonse, our priest from Dallas, to officiate at our wedding. Even though he was an hour late to the rehearsal the night before, he stood on time at the front of the church and greeted Eric and me with the warmest smile. His words were very eloquent. He described Eric and me as a holy and wild couple. *Wild?* For sure, we were embarking on a wild ride. The service was beautiful. It was surreal to see and hear every detail become reality: each song sung, each chosen reading spoken, and every word of our vows shared face to face in front of family and friends. When I looked out at the congregation, I was in awe of all our loved ones who traveled to be with us. I loved seeing the fascinators worn so stylishly de rigueur by the women who traveled from England and

Ireland. The service was finally made complete when Father Alfonse announced it was time for the groom to kiss his bride.

Hallelujah!!! We were finally Mr. and Mrs. Kuban!!!

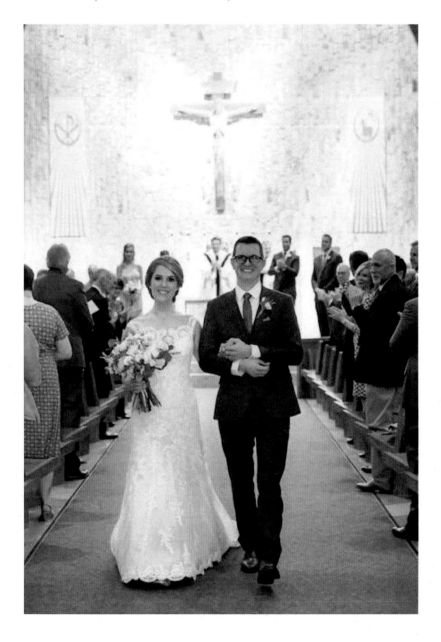

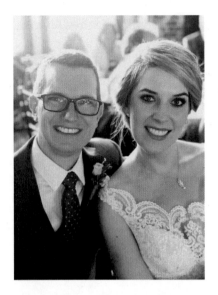
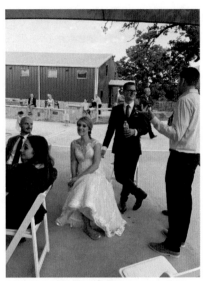
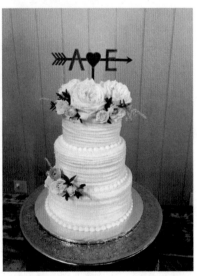
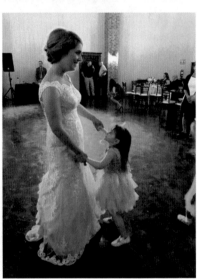

The reception was held at the Broken Arrow Ranch outside Bryan. It was gratifying to see the realization after all the details that Eric and I had planned together for entertaining our family and friends. The party barn was decorated Texas-chic with flowers and succulents, and the atmosphere was joyous. Following the introduction of bridesmaids, groomsmen, and

Jack, the ring-bearer, the DJ introduced for the first time, Mr. and Mrs. Kuban. I held my bouquet above my head with one hand and my husband's hand with the other as we walked into the room to the clamor of applauding guests. Eric and I were seated at the head table and bowed our heads for the blessing before the traditional Texas BBQ dinner with all the trimmings. Our plates were brought to the table as if we were royalty. I certainly felt like a princess. I don't think I was able to eat much, but I was primarily afraid of dropping BBQ sauce on my white wedding dress.

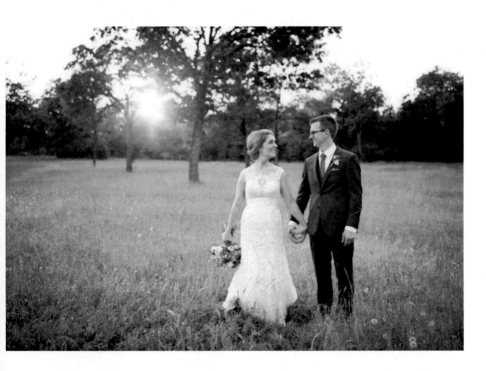

As guests finished eating, the music coaxed them to the dance floor. I had planned a special moment for our last dance. I wanted to mark the moment with a surprise for Eric. Slipping away to the bridal suite where I had dressed for the wedding, I stood in front of the mirror and removed my wig.

Eric gasped when he walked into the room. He grabbed my hands and, with tears in his eyes, told me I was beautiful. I could feel my heart beating as a lump in my throat; much like the time that I removed my beanie for

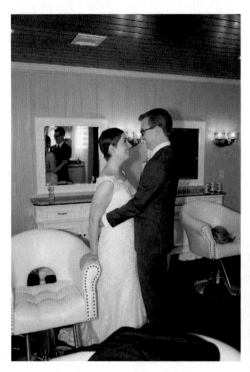

the first time to reveal my bald head for Eric to see. He told me then that I was beautiful. This time, with my blonde wig thrown in a chair, I was sporting a short, brunette pixie cut. The symbolism of my authentic look was transparent in how much I could feel the pride that Eric had in me at that exposed moment.

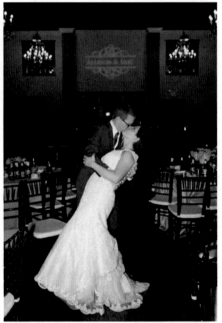

Eric and I held hands firmly as the DJ re-introduced us as the NEW Mr. and Mrs. Kuban. As we entered the dance floor, everyone was rising, standing on chairs, and taking photos. My eyes caught my mom and dad, uncles, and aunts in tears as they watched our solo dance. When the tempo of the song quickened, Eric twirled me around to **She's Like Texas** and

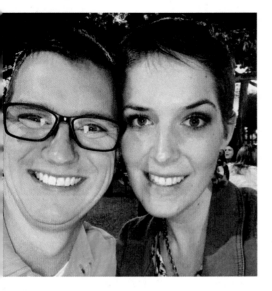

everyone cheered as he dipped me low and held me strongly in his arms. There was no worry of the wig falling at an inopportune moment. I felt very secure.

We left the reception with a sparkler sendoff. After hours of intense emotions and activity, Eric and I had a silent moment together while being driven to the hotel. While I had held myself together by sheer force of will all day, that queasy, nauseous feeling hit me. *Dammit, not on my wedding night.* In the hotel room, Eric helped unhook the many buttons on the back of my dress. All the while, I was praying to myself, *please let me be a normal wife tonight.* To be brief (and respectful), we fulfilled the best first night of our lives as Mr. and Mrs. Kuban.

When I woke up in the morning after the excitement of our wonderful wedding day and a nauseous night in the bathroom, I was drained. We had a family brunch to attend that Sunday morning. I dressed and did not wear my wig. At the brunch, everyone told me how proud they were and how much they loved my short pixie cut. My dad told me it was the end of the era as I embraced this new hairdo. Despite this being a wonderful morning and a perfect way to hug my loved ones before we left for our honeymoon, I was weak and nauseous, excusing myself to go to the bathroom every few minutes. I desperately wanted to lay down. Looking at the brunch food just added to my nausea. My new father-in-law brought me Gatorade and ordered a prescription of Zofran for me; a fitting farewell gift as Eric and I departed for the Texas Hill Country. Getting started on the three-hour car ride with my new husband, I was praying that we would find restrooms along the way.

My stomach bug slowly eased. Our honeymoon was both restful and adventuresome. We kept it simple, unlike our lives over the past several months. It was a pleasure staying in B&Bs, enjoying springtime in Texas with the wildflowers, and perfect weather. We walked around Fredericksburg, checked out shops, ate fabulous meals, hiked to the top of Enchanted Rock, and had romantic dinners with just enough wine to feel confident in the lingerie that my friends had bought me for my bachelorette party just one month earlier.

With increased stamina, I could stay up later and enjoy special moments with my husband. I was feeling my old self again. I was happy and felt good. Even a phone call from my new boss at the hotel could not spoil my mood. He had a question that I had specifically answered in my notes before leaving. My friend Toya, the assistant general manager, had my back. She couldn't believe that I was interrupted on my honeymoon. I put the call out of mind; I would be back in the office soon enough.

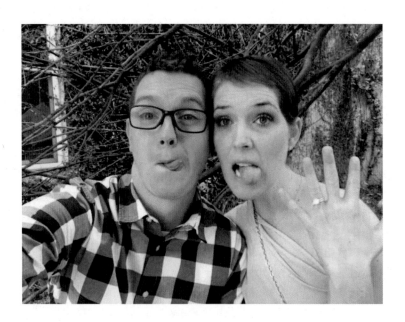

SOMETHINGS GOTTA GIVE

Returning to Dallas after the honeymoon, I dreaded going back to work. Sadly, that dread lived up to my worst expectations. My time at work through the summer of 2018 was really tough. The job became more and more demanding as the new management company insisted on reinventing the wheel over and over. Programs changed every other day. Passwords to programs never worked. The staff was frustrated and quitting. The management company needed more and more from me, while providing little support from corporate. I was mustering energy from a perpetually drained body.

When not at work, I was at home trying to be a wife to Eric. Our work schedules rarely matched up. He would be away for days at a time with his irregular schedule. When I was home, I had little energy. I became more and more stressed. My coping mechanisms became increasingly unhealthy. I was gaining weight and becoming uncomfortable with my body. I became more depressed. I was unhappy with work, lonely when Eric wasn't home, anxious that I couldn't perform at work, or be the wife I wanted to be. I was on a downward spiral. I was hating the reality that I had created. I wanted to go back to chemo. I wanted the feeling of being so drugged up that I didn't have to face my own reality. I wanted to escape.

I was well aware that LOXO-292, the trial medicine, was saving my life. Going for staging scans over the past few months made me anxious. Even "stable" results made me anxious. I had a scan in May at MD Anderson. This time, my doctor came into the room with the news that my tumors had shrunk 38 percent! My dad, mom, and Eric were in tears. The hope that I saw in their faces gave me the will to keep going.

The excitement from Dr. Subbiah as he shared this news reassured me that I was on the right path. The confidence he showed back in January was evident again as he said, "I told you this would work."

Around this time, my family signed up to participate in the Purple Stride Pancreatic Cancer Walk in Houston. As a survivor, I was recognized and was invited on stage with other survivors to be recognized. "Hi I'm Allison Kuban and I have been a survivor for 11 months."

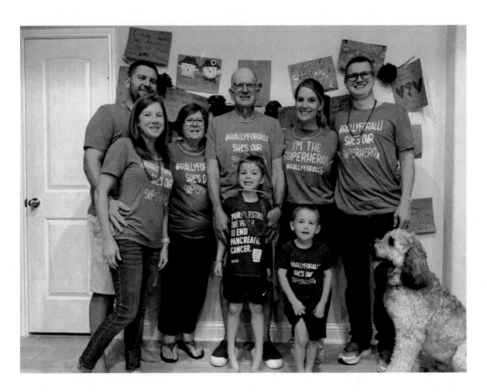

The moment seemed surreal; others spoke of surviving several years or several weeks. A fellow survivor told his story to the crowd. He gave me hope that my story might touch someone someday.

I needed that weekend. I needed that hope to bring me back to my new reality. *Alli, you have a great life and have been given a second chance.*

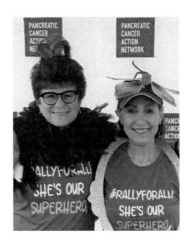

The boost that I got from the Purple Stride event was short-lived when I returned to work in Dallas. Anxiety set in and I found myself taking Xanax in anticipation of facing the day. This became a daily occurrence. My old normal work ethic was so far out of reach. I could no longer pull the 12-hour days or employ the systems that I could once do in my sleep. The work was taking its toll on my mind, body, and spirit. Each day wore me out to the point where I had nothing to give to other areas of my life, primarily my health and my marriage. While trying to prove to everyone that I was in control of my work-life balance, I was losing myself.

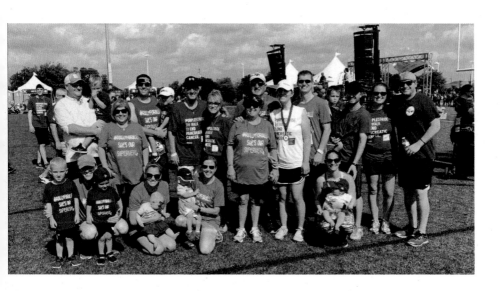

DESPERATE TIMES, DESPERATE MEASURES

I turned to food and Xanax as coping mechanisms. As my health increased and stress rose, my weight increased. My self-image plummeted. I became more depressed and could feel myself becoming a ticking time bomb with every incoming email, phone call, or meeting being a potential detonator. I felt the veins in my forehead pulsating. I suppressed all my emotions until it was too much. I did not enjoy a hug or kiss from Eric. I was lost. I would cry to the point where I couldn't breathe because crying felt better than the suffocating feeling I experienced with the stress and anxiety.

I was so unhappy.

All I could think of was how easy my life had been just a few months earlier. I missed the attentive nurses during my treatments, my family being around me every day, and the legitimate excuse for being absent from work. Perhaps, more frightening, I missed the feeling of euphoria from all the medications that kept me sedated. I was desperate for freedom from my own thoughts.

In my desperation, I grew angry and contemplated stopping my medicine without telling anyone. By self-inflicting harm, I could escape how unhappy I was. I felt like a failure. I wanted to fail. And I wanted to die.

Eric had no knowledge of my suicidal thoughts until I finally confided in him at a monthly appointment. He paced the room, throwing his hands up and down, covering his face in disbelief. He had so much hope for me and our future but saw that I was throwing it away. When I told Eric how desperate and depressed I was, he said he could no longer help me and I needed an intervention or therapist to help us.

This was my lowest point. I felt empty. Seeing the look of despair on Eric's face, I promised to never toy with my medication and asked him to keep this episode just between us. I promised to make an appointment with the oncology psychologist at UT Southwestern when we returned to Dallas.

As promised, I made the call and was referred to a doctor who specializes in psychology for cancer patients. While waiting for this new doctor, I recognized the room across the hall from where I used to wait for my infusions. Memories of the taste of saline filled my mouth. When my name was called, I was greeted by a beautiful lady with a welcoming smile. At that session, she heard about all my pent-up stresses such as planning the wedding, coming down from the emotional high, facing a new management company, feeling unappreciated and undervalued at my work place, trying to live a normal loving life with my new husband, and going through the emotions and changes from my illness. She recognized from my tear-stained face that something needed to give. I met with her two other times and my stress and anxiety never seemed to improve. My level of stress was unhealthy and she recommended I make a change. My marriage and my health were the most important things and I needed to focus on them. Everything else had to wait.

Eric and I decided on a solution together. After so much time and energy spent in my hotel management career, it was a painful decision to leave my job. The job had defined me for so long. It was hard to leave my co-workers, the friends who became like family. Despite the animosity I felt toward the new management company, it was hard to walk away from a career that I built after four years of university and ten years of professional experiences. *What was I supposed to say when people asked me what I do?* This is a question that would continue to haunt me for years.

I turned in my two-weeks' notice. I prepared my staff for my final departure, filled open positions, and left my successor with passwords and my well wishes and hopes for great success. I walked out those hotel front doors one last time, as an unemployed woman and immediately felt an identity crisis.

SHE'S GOT THOSE SUMMERTIME BLUES

In the summer of 2018, as I was gaining my physical strength back, my mental health continued to deteriorate. *How do I fix the constant heartache and nagging voice in my brain that a "normal life" will not exist anymore?*

Isolation and uncertainty haunted me. Meeting people, particularly new people, gave me anxiety. *Who was I?* I did not have a career. I did not have children. I had cancer. But I did not look like a cancer patient; my body was gaining strength and had the appearance of a healthy woman. I found myself having to repeat over and over that I had cancer. That was my identity. I was becoming self-conscious about this identity. I preferred isolation rather than explanation.

At this time, I could not make sense of this renewed chance at life through a new experimental drug. Here I was, getting physically stronger. I should go out and conquer the world, but just making it through each day was challenging enough. Cancer was no longer holding me back physically, but it was dominating my identity, my thoughts, and my relationships. No treatment protocols or discharge instructions offered any guidance for this part of my healing. The way forward was blinded by my anxiety and depression.

When people asked how I felt, it was easier to tell them that I was doing great. *I am conquering cancer and persevering. I am beating all the odds.* Now that this victory was becoming secure, I should have wisdom, strength, and a new appreciation for life. However, I felt anything but that. Messages from the Rally for Alli group reminded me that I could "move mountains" and be a "pioneer for health." All of this made me internalize the person I thought I should be and wanted to be. *What if just waking up to breathe and not take a handful of pills to calm side effects was enough?*

By leaving my job in order to focus on myself, I lost myself even further. I had become so distant from that person who I had been pre-cancer diagnosis that I could not stand to look at this stranger in the mirror. Rather than face the psychological demons that haunted me, it was easier to lie and say I was okay, then fantasize about being sick and careless again.

In my life's journey, I had arrived at the exact opposite place from what I had mapped out. I went from an adventure-seeking, goal-setting, accomplishment-driven woman to a withdrawn, anxious, fearful person. Feelings of survivor's guilt compounded my shame. I was lucky to be alive when so many people that I love were not. My friend Danielle, who was a pillar of strength during my initial chemo days, succumbed to her disease after her breast cancer metastasized to her skin. Out of the numerous people that I met through the pancreatic cancer groups, I had outlasted so many.

TIME TO REFRESH THE FAIRY TALE

Once upon a time...

... there was a princess who was ambitious in her career and love of life. Although she put dating on hold until her 30th birthday, she still harbored the dreams of becoming a wife and mother. She loved to travel and to meet up with friends and family for holidays and parties. She envisioned a once upon a time with her prince charming.

Like most fairy tales, there is a dashing prince who stole the young princess' heart with a kiss and a promise of eternal love. However, the fairy tale turned frightful. Not with a prick of a spinning wheel needle or bite of a poison apple, but an ache that lurked in her body and wreaked havoc on her heart and soul. The princess was lost in a bleak forest with no visible paths to return to her happy place.

On a bright side, the fairy tale had a conjurer with great powers who mixed and tested a potion that had magical potency and gave hope to the princess even when she couldn't smile at times.

There was a super friendly village where the sun always shone and birds chirped a cheery melody. The village was full of lovely people who kept vigil over the princess and lifted her low spirits when times got rough for her ...

THE WAY FORWARD

Oh my, how I wanted the fairy tale life to end "happily ever after".

Recovering from cancer or, if you are lucky, learning to live with it, is not a gentle course. The scars and memories will linger. For me, it is not about salvaging who I was but accepting the path I have been given. Recreating oneself can be terrifying when you felt like you were on top at one point and at the bottom-most depths the next.

My beginning anew was full of anxiety and panic attacks that left me gulping for my next breath. Even positive changes in my body evoked a haunting feeling that this miraculous concoction of medical marvel was at work in ways that are still a mystery to me. The longing for motherhood brings on deeply buried emotions that resurface when I see mothers pushing their children in strollers and building a future for them.

One might say I had reasons for being depressed, but there was still a part of my being that told me to "snap out of it." I had a choice to (1) live my life

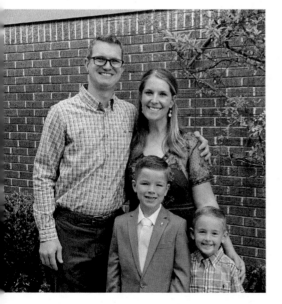

being happy or (2) dwell on my anxiety and fear. Eric helped me to focus on the things that brought us together: love of travel, love of family, love of Christ, love for each other, and so much more.

Eric has been my rock and support for all decisions that affect my health and happiness. We made the decision to move from Dallas to Houston to be closer to Andrew, Miranda, Jack and Ben, and my medical team at MD Anderson. Being in close proximity to family continues to lift my spirits, particularly since Eric can be away from home for days at a time with work. Eric and I bought a home just two blocks from my brother and his family. They include me in tons of activities, sporting events for the kids, and even mom's nights out with friends.

Watching our nephews grow is a lovely, heart-filling alternative to not raising our own children. This move offered a new beginning for Eric and me. We accepted the profound disappointment knowing we would not have our own children but could cherish the love and time spent with our nephews. Being aunt and uncle is of utmost importance in our lives; strengthening our relationship as husband and wife. That renewed strength has made it possible for us to continue our adventures by traveling to Cuba, Japan, and a return to France where we had our first international trip before this story of survival started.

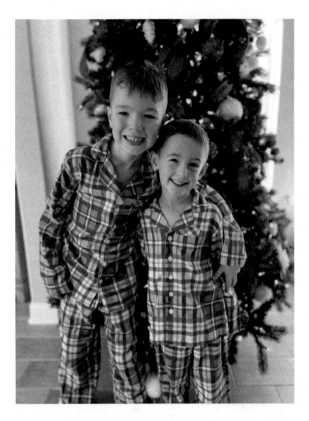

The rock-solid guarantee that the final chapter will have a happily ever after scenario is the enduring love story between the princess and the noble prince. Eric was "that guy" who called me at the wrong time before I turned 30. The truth is that Eric came into my life at just the exact moment that he was needed. I thought my life was planned out with a career, marriage, and children. Eric had similar plans. His hopes and dreams for his future changed as mine changed. Eric proved to be the adventurous traveler that I dreamed of sharing my life with. Even when the adventure took a surprise turn, he was at my bedside as I fought for life. Eric was part of the drug trial by keeping the faith when I had none.

Moving forward is the only way to go. Every moment, big and small, is part of our love story. Eric is the knight in shining armor by my side, in sickness and in health, and second chances. Eric helps me remember to seek more in life. On my 32nd birthday Eric surprised me with an unexpected jump from an airplane. He took me rock climbing. I have learned to be open to new adventures at home and in the community. Eric encourages me to volunteer and share my story of hope with strangers. He reminds me that we have one life to live and gives me once in a lifetime experiences to help fill my mind and heart as I keep moving forward.

Eric shares with me the painful conversations about parenthood through natural childbirth that is not in our future. He reminds me to focus on what we do have, our family and each other.

What if this path in life is better than the one I had planned?

REMEMBERING DANIELLE AND HEATHER

As several friends succumbed to the cancer, I kept finding myself asking: *Why me? Why do I get this second chance? What is my purpose?*

When Danielle, my friend and colleague who worked with me in Orlando, passed away a few years ago, I was still in the midst of my initial fight with pancreatic cancer. Death was foreshadowing. I feared every hospital visit for a staging scan. When my narrative changed for the better, I began sharing my hope with others.

My friend Heather was diagnosed with an aggressive form of adenocarcinoma. The cancer was in her stomach lining and spread to her brain. We often talked about the reasons why we were given this battle and both felt solace that our experiences would help another cancer patient someday. Heather was placed on hospice. Eric flew to Salt Lake City with me so that I could be with her once again. I laid beside her and shared hope as we held hands in her final hours. Heather passed away just a week later. Her passing shook me to the core. I felt like it was an even bigger mission to share not just my hope, but hers.

After Heather's death, her sister, Holly, called to let me know her genetic testing matched with the same gene that Heather had. Holly's scan detected cancer in her stomach. The cancer detection was caught early and Holly was scheduled for surgery to remove her stomach. If it weren't for Heather's battle, Holly and many others would not have known to be tested and look for this same gene found in Heather's cancer cells.

Genomic profiling is how doctors found my mutation. I truly wish this would be a standard procedure for detecting potential cancers in patients. Fortunately, more and more scientists, researchers, and doctors are turning to it as they see successes. Heather's story ultimately had a successful chapter, even though the ending was not what we hoped for.

TAKE ONE EXIT AT A TIME

I attribute a conscious awakening point to something I read in **Between Two Kingdoms: A Memoir of a Life Interrupted** by Suleika Jaouad.

> *"What if I stopped thinking of pain as something that needs to be numbed, fixed, dodged, and protected against? What if I tried to honor its presence in my body to welcome it as a part of life?"*

Suleika had been given a 35% chance of survival from leukemia. After almost four years of treatments that took a huge toll on her mental and physical health, Suleika was considered cured of her cancer. She relapsed in July 2022.

Was I wrong to think that "healing" meant ridding my body of the pain and illness? Could I truly leave all the pain and ailing behind me?

I began to learn from Suleika that this is not how it works. Healing is figuring out how to coexist with the pain and the tumor that still clings to my pancreas. It is very possible that my cancer will always be a part of my body. Accepting my experience with cancer was the first step in healing.

Accepting to grieve the woman that I was before the diagnosis was hard, perhaps the hardest part of the acceptance process. I was scared that the pre-diagnosed Alli was who everyone expected to emerge again. I grieved for Allison at 29½ years old. I struggled to move on from what had happened and find a new purpose for my life.

I have realized that I don't actually need to grieve for this loss. The past years of yo-yo health is not meant to be lost and not something to forget. In fact, I don't want to forget. These experiences and memories, good and often miserable, are a huge part of the woman I am today. I have steadily learned that this is my story of resilience and hope.

The expectations of a happily ever after chapter to this story are bright and may take a lifetime to complete. I will be working on myself every day. I acknowledge the power of prayer sustained me over the years, as well as a profound respect for the advancement of medical science. This story will always be made richer with the frequent appearance of family and friends. The Rally for Alli Facebook gives a virtual presence online.

I began sharing my story with a new outlook. I was featured in MD Anderson's medical journals, on PanCan's survivor stories, and in several news interviews. I have been given opportunities to further advocate for

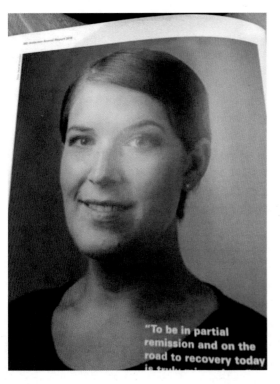

"To be in partial remission and on the road to recovery today

medical research. Imagine the time when you may have been asked about the future. *What would you do if you could make one dream come true? Did you answer, find a cure for cancer?* I am living that dream on the trial drug. I hope that by advocating more and more about the success of this one trial drug, additional money will go to research for every type of cancer and that dream will become a reality for everyone.

In April 2022, I was asked to speak at the Houston Cattle Baron's Ball, a major fundraiser in support of the American Cancer Society. The resources and impact of the American Cancer Society are boundless; including research and patient support during treatment and when in remission. These are points I wanted to emphasize from my speech.

Cancer knocked me down. But it also built me up. If asked for advice, I say you must be your own advocate and learn to trust the advice of experts and a supportive family. You have to find the doctors that are HOPEFUL and support YOU in your journey.

How did I get directed to targeted therapy and find a doctor who believed in it? I had a family who encouraged me to be brave. They stayed hopeful, even if I was starting to question it. And even though my doctor did tell me that 99% of the time the testing comes back without a clear answer, I was that 1% who just might beat the odds.

I've experienced survivor's guilt after meeting so many people who have succumbed to their diseases. I know the feeling of loss. I grieve the old Alli and the future that she had planned. But I know, in this moment, this is where I should be. Using my voice to advocate for research and support.

Unfortunately, pancreatic cancer is hard to detect and is often found when it's too late. That's why we hear of so many people with pancreatic cancer dying very quickly after the initial diagnosis. However, in the past 5 years since I've been fighting this health hurdle, the 5-year survival rate has gone up from 8% to 11%. On my 36th birthday in June 2022, I will officially be a part of this statistic. And I'll be damned if I don't see it go up another percentage.

WHAT DOES THE FUTURE HOLD? HOLD ON!

As I approached my 36th birthday, I was excited to find out LOXO-292, my trial drug, was up for approval by the Food and Drug Administration. I felt validated, triumphant, and part of medical history. It was my hope that Jack and Ben would know the hope that I bring to a cancer diagnosis rather than the fear of it.

As my 5-year survival anniversary approached that June, I was excited for the future. I felt like that would be a moment in time where a significant chapter in life would close and a new one begins.

However, a month before this milestone, history had an unexpected way of repeating itself. When I told my doctor about experiencing dizzy spells, he ordered a brain scan. I thought it was a bit excessive but went ahead with it. To put it briefly, I was diagnosed with a malignant neoplasm of the brain (aka brain tumor).

Fortunately, Dr. Subbiah was aware that this could be a possibility, and the tumor was detected early. With the trial, I had been under a microscope at MD Anderson with my medical history meticulously tracked. He assured me this brain cancer was a "hiccup" and we should press forward. His confidence in me over the past five years did not waver in this moment.

The treatment plan for this hiccup was Gamma Knife Radiation. It was a one-time radiation treatment that was not invasive. The recovery time was expected to be a couple of days. However, the following few months were extremely difficult as I faced numerous challenges.

I found myself dwelling in familiar anxiety and depression as I watched my body change, yet again, from the medicines I was taking. I suffered from extreme headaches, brain pressure and general discomfort. I was unable to enjoy the usual daily things that I had begun to get used to. I couldn't exercise, couldn't take care of the house, and couldn't play with my nephews. I pushed Eric away, fearing for him to go through a caregiving role, yet again with me. But he stayed by my side, reassuring me that we had done this before and can do it again.

The overwhelming thoughts pounding inside my head and the recurring depression took a toll. I sought relief and ended up self-medicating with Zoloft. However, the Zoloft mixed with my other medicines, had an adverse reaction. I ended up in the ICU on a ventilator with Serotonin Syndrome.

When I woke up and realized what was happening, I was sickened at the thought of Eric and my parents seeing me lay helpless in the hospital bed. I went from writing my to-do lists to barely scribbling the words, "Am I going to die?" on a white board that I was forced to use since I couldn't speak with the endotracheal tube.

Also on my mind, Jack and Ben were five years older since my first cancer diagnosis and could reason, think for themselves, and express feelings. *What do the boys think about Auntie Alli? Why can't we go to her house and do crafts and play games?* The worst feeling was that I let down my Rally for Alli community. All these people had witnessed a miracle and celebrated my survival over the past five years. I was embarrassed and fearful of what people would think of me. *Did she overdose on drugs? Is she mentally unstable? Why is her face and neck so puffy?*

However, the doctors would not let me fail. My family would not let me fail. Eric would not let me fail.

I spent the next several months in therapy and regaining my strength both physically and mentally. I had to accept what happened but not let it define me. I reread that portion of Suleika's book and decided to seek a therapist to help me move past the trauma.

FINDING THE NEEDLE IN THE HAYSTACK

In the time since my trial started, Eli Lilly acquired Loxo Oncology, the company that created LOXO-292. In the spring of 2022, I was introduced to Devon, a representative from Eli Lilly. I quickly became a real person with a name, not just the longest line on their bar graph with pancreatic cancer. Previously, I was only a statistic that showed the positive results they were hoping for and working hard to achieve. Devon was enthusiastic about the Eli Lilly facilities and researchers for the drug that I have been taking for 4+ years.

In September 2022, my phone buzzed with a text message from Devon, "Thank you for being part of this research. It was approved." My heart skipped a beat. The drug would now be available to the public and was released by the name Retevmo (selpercatinib).

Dr. Subbiah called to thank me for trusting him. This man, who had so much confidence in me four years ago when I came in with a sweater cap covering a bald head and sweats hanging loosely from a barely 110-pound body, called to say thank you. His trust in this trial and in me had come to a hopeful fruition. I felt a true feeling of accomplishment. Dr. Subbiah had always told me about this search for survival and I was "a needle in a haystack."

That search for the needle took 4+ years. My survival at the hands of medical miracles and powerful prayers resulted in exposing that bright shiny needle. I am a survivor and I helped make it possible for many patients who follow to make that same claim. The needle may have just become a bit easier to find in the haystack.

EPILOGUE

It was my original intention for this book to focus on the years from my initial diagnosis in June 2017 until June 2022, which would mark the fifth milestone year.

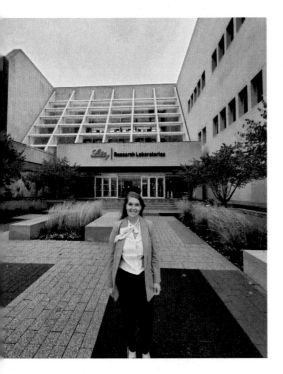

But you cannot always plan for the ways that cancer may course through your body. In June 2022, just when I planned to celebrate that milestone in my recovery, I was diagnosed with another form of cancer, a malignant neoplasm of the brain. This second bout with cancer proved to be more of a mental game.

Thankfully, I already had the tools necessary to overcome the shock of a new setback. I recognized my weaknesses and allowed myself to embrace them. I had learned to be a strong warrior against cancer and entered this second battle with that mindset.

Over the fall of 2022, I was returning to some normalcy and started to enjoy things in life that had previously brought me joy. This good news came with more good news. Eli Lilly invited me to Indianapolis for a Town Hall, visit the bottling plant, and meet the researchers who developed the formula that reacted with RET fusion. This became the experimental drug, that made its way to MD Anderson for clinical trials, that landed in the palm of my hand to swallow twice a day, that gave me a new life.

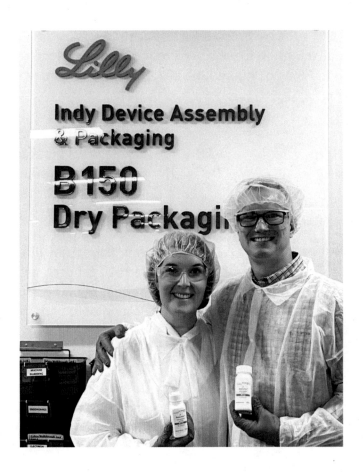

Meeting the team at Eli Lilly was a full circle moment in my cancer journey. I was able to look these men and women in the eye, face to face. They could see me as a walking, breathing example of the success of their medical ingenuity. As much as I was in awe of their accomplishments, they were in awe of my story that I shared. They were the life-saving superheroes who made possible a reality that allows me to share hope.

This book has been a glimpse of a very short, very dramatic period of my life.

This Is Not The End.

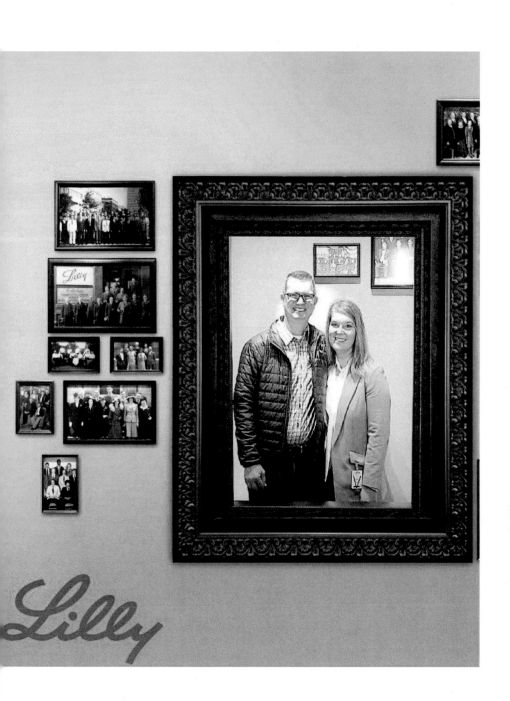

Made in the USA
Columbia, SC
25 February 2023

1b66dc55-2713-43c3-91ba-cbf7697c695fR01